# Spurgeon's Color Atlas of
## Large Animal Anatomy:
### *The Essentials*

# Spurgeon's Color Atlas of
# Large Animal Anatomy:
## *The Essentials*

## Thomas O. McCracken, MS
*Former Associate Professor of Anatomy*
*College of Veterinary Medicine and Biomedical Sciences*
*Colorado State University*
*Vice President for Product and Development*
*Visible Productions LLC*
*Fort Collins, Colorado*

## Robert A. Kainer, DVM, MS
*Professor Emeritus of Anatomy*
*College of Veterinary Medicine and Biomedical Sciences*
*Colorado State University*
*Fort Collins, Colorado*

## Thomas L. Spurgeon, PhD
*Late Associate Professor of Anatomy*
*College of Veterinary Medicine and Biomedical Sciences*
*Colorado State University*
*Fort Collins, Colorado*

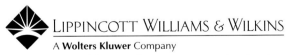

### LIPPINCOTT WILLIAMS & WILKINS
A **Wolters Kluwer** Company

Philadelphia · Baltimore · New York · London
Buenos Aires · Hong Kong · Sydney · Tokyo

*Editor:* Donna Balado
*Managing Editor:* Crystal Taylor
*Marketing Manager:* Jennifer Conrad
*Production Editor:* Karen Ruppert

Copyright © 1999 Lippincott Williams & Wilkins

351 West Camden Street
Baltimore, Maryland 21201-2436 USA

530 Walnut Street,
Philadelphia, Pennsylvania 19106-3621

*Printed in the United States of America*
First Edition

**Library of Congress Cataloging-in-Publication Data**

McCracken, Thomas O.
   Spurgeon's color atlas of large animal anatomy : the essentials /
Thomas O. McCracken, Robert A. Kainer, Thomas L. Spurgeon
     p.  cm.
   ISBN 0-683-30673-1
   1. Veterinary anatomy Atlases.    I. Kainer, Robert A.    II. Title.
SF76l.M35  1999
636.089'1--dc2l                  99-20525
                                CIP

*The publishers have made every effort to trace the copyright holders for borrowed material. If they have inadvertently overlooked any, they will be pleased to make the necessary arrangements at the first opportunity.*

To purchase additional copies of this book, call our customer service department at **(800) 638-3030** or fax orders to **(301) 824-7390**. International customers should call **(301) 714-2324**.

00 01 02 03
2 3 4 5 6 7 8 9 10

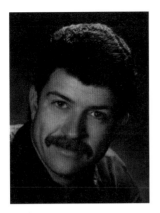

*Thomas Spurgeon*

## TO OUR COLLEAGUE AND FRIEND

*Dr. Thomas L. Spurgeon, exceptionally well-trained anatomist, superb teacher, and educational innovator, devoted his professional life to the advancement of anatomic education through scientific investigation and the dissemination of anatomic knowledge.*

*Following service to his country in the United States Air Force, Thomas L. Spurgeon entered college. Upon completion of his doctorate in anatomy in the School of Veterinary Medicine at the University of California-Davis, Dr. Spurgeon accepted a faculty position in the College of Veterinary Medicine at Washington State University. His record as an excellent anatomist at that institution led to a position in the College of Veterinary Medicine and Biomedical Sciences at Colorado State University.*

*His broad knowledge of both human and veterinary anatomy was utilized fully at Colorado State. Students requiring courses in basic human anatomy as well as those majoring in veterinary medicine and various animal sciences profited from the instruction provided by this well-rounded anatomist who possessed outstanding pedagogic skill. His expertise was equally appreciated by the graduate students he mentored, particularly those in the biomedical illustration program.*

*Dr. Spurgeon, a pioneer in the computer-assisted instruction of anatomy, was continually seeking new methods of presentation. He and his colleague and close friend, Thomas O. McCracken, conceived the unique anatomic presentation used in this atlas.*

*Tragically, Dr. Spurgeon's untimely death in an automobile accident in 1997 brought a halt to his brilliant career. Dr. Spurgeon's devoted sons, Aaron and Kyle, are indeed proud of their father's accomplishments. Countless students mourn the passing of a man who, as teacher and friend, contributed so much to their lives.*

# ACKNOWLEDGMENTS

Many talented individuals contributed to the production of *Spurgeon's Color Atlas of Large Animal Anatomy: The Essentials.* Foremost among them were the artists, Conery Calhoon, Molly Babich, Gale Mueller, and Sandra Mullins, who colored Thomas McCracken's original drawings of anatomic specimens. They employed manual and digital techniques to reproduce the subtle colors of tissues and organs.

Consultants, who authored plates drawn by Thomas McCracken, selected clinical conditions and husbandry applications based on their anatomic significance. The consultants were Dr. Gayle Trotter for the horse; Dr. Frank Garry for the ox; Dr. Joan Bowen for the sheep and goat; Dr. LaRue Johnson for the llama and alpaca and the swine; and Dr. John Avens for the chicken. These specialists reviewed the plates on the various species, enhancing the accuracy of the presentations. Their contributions are gratefully acknowledged.

Carroll Cann, Executive Editor of Teton-New Media, was an enthusiastic supporter of the concept of the atlas. We thank him for his suggestions and encouragement.

Special thanks are due the late Dr. Patricia Brooks who supported her husband, Dr. Spurgeon, and frequently assisted him in his work. She, too, was a contributor to this atlas.

We greatly appreciated the reliable assistance of Dennis Madden, pathology technician in the College of Veterinary Medicine and Biomedical Sciences at Colorado State University. His procurement of specimens and his dissection skills were essential to the production of this atlas.

We thank Mark Goldstein for a student's viewpoint. His assistance with compilation of the index and his review and comments on the plates were most helpful.

We are grateful to Dr. Michael Smith from the School of Veterinary Medicine at Ross University for his careful review of the final proofs. His knowledge of anatomy, his fine teaching skills, and his critical eye well qualified him for this arduous task.

Acknowledgment is due the Department of Anatomy and Neurobiology and the Department of Clinical Sciences at Colorado State University for the use of their facilities and for providing living animals, skeletons, embalmed specimens, and necropsy specimens. Dr. Robert Lee prepared and was most helpful in providing anatomic specimens. We acknowledge the kindness of exhibitors at the National Western Stock Show and Midnight Valley Friesens for permission to photograph their animals.

We thank Alpine Publications, Inc. of Loveland, Colorado, for permission to use drawings from our book, *Horse Anatomy, A Coloring Atlas.* Permission from Pfizer Animal Health Group to use drawings of the chicken's anatomy from *Anatomical Atlas* is also appreciated.

# CONTENTS

## SECTION 1    THE HORSE *(Equus caballus)*

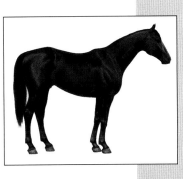

## SECTION 2    THE OX *(Bos taurus,* also *Bos indicus)*

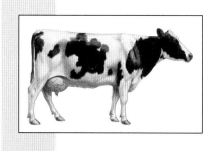

## SECTION 3  THE SHEEP *(Ovis aries)*

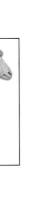

## SECTION 4  THE GOAT *(Capra hircus)*

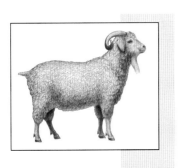

## SECTION 5    THE LLAMA AND ALPACA *(Lama glama and Lama pacos)*

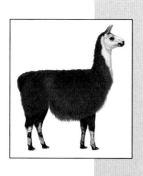

## SECTION 6    THE SWINE *(Sus scrofa domesticus)*

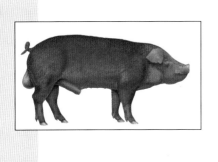

## SECTION 7    THE CHICKEN (*Gallus gallus domesticus*)

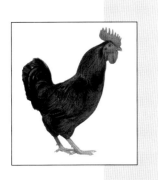

# INTRODUCTION

S *purgeon's Color Atlas of Large Animal Anatomy: The Essentials* is not a complete, detailed anatomic atlas. Instead, it presents topographic relationships of the major organs of the horse, ox, sheep, goat, llama, alpaca (a smaller species with long, lustrous hair), swine, and chicken in a simple yet technically accurate format. As an important food animal, the chicken is included with the large domestic animals in this atlas. Throughout the *Atlas,* most male and female of a given species are on facing pages. The majority of the plates contain information on the entire body. Some plates are confined to a region; a few contain organs isolated from the rest of the body. Whereas most systems (e.g., digestive and reproductive) are presented for each animal, other systems are included only for some species to illustrate general anatomic patterns. Structures common to the various animals are labeled several times; other structures are labeled on only one or two species, usually emphasizing specific anatomy (the anatomy peculiar to a certain species). Animal specialists authored plates illustrating selected clinical or husbandry applications that reflect the anatomy of the organs involved.

The *Atlas* is intended for use by individuals at different stages of their education, serving as a survey of the specific anatomy of the different animals. Advanced 4-H club members, high school vocational agriculture students, and college students studying veterinary medical technology, veterinary medicine, animal science, and wildlife biology can use this *Atlas* as an introduction to the anatomy of common farm animals. The *Atlas* can also serve as a reference for horse breeders and trainers, as well as livestock and poultry producers. It will provide a quick review for persons with previous training in anatomy and will be an invaluable aid for the professional—e.g., a veterinarian or animal scientist—in explaining to a client some aspect of anatomy that pertains to an animal's condition and needs.

The following introductory pages provide the reader with a background in nomenclature and anatomic orientation.

# NOMENCLATURE AND ANATOMIC ORIENTATION

## ANIMAL CLASSIFICATION

The horse (*Equus caballus*) is classified as an odd-toed ungulate (hoofed mammal) in the order Perissodactyla, suborder Hippomorpha, and family Equidae. Members of this family are termed equids. "Equine" is an adjective. Equine characteristics include the grouping of limb muscles close to the trunk with tendons extending over long third metacarpal and metatarsal bones to the digits, providing leverage for sustained, rapid locomotion. Because this leverage arrangement does not develop great force, the heavy draft horse must rely on body weight to perform pulling tasks. Another equine characteristic is the horse's extensive large intestine, the site of final microbial digestion and absorption of nutrients.

Cloven-hoofed ungulates that walk on their third and fourth digits are in the order Artiodactyla. Domestic ungulates in the suborder Ruminantia include those in the family Bovidae, subfamily Bovinae—the ox (*Bos taurus*) and zebu (*Bos indicus*)—and subfamily caprinae, the sheep (*Ovis aries*) and goat (*Capra hircus*). The noun "bovids" (after Bovidae) is usually reserved for cattle, bison, yak, and water buffalo; sheep are ovids and goats are caprids, named according to each genus. Adjectives end in -ine: bovine, ovine, and caprine, respectively.

The llama (*Lama glama*) and alpaca (*Lama pacos*) are cud-chewing artiodactyls from South America called camelids, named after the family Camelidae in the suborder Tylopoda. South American camelids are also called lamoids. Both ruminants and camelids have large, compartmented stomachs essential for the microbial digestion of cellulose. Feed is more finely divided by rumination, a physiologic sequence of regurgitation of stomach contents, remastication (chewing), and redeglutition (swallowing).

Swine (pigs are young; hogs are mature) are artiodactyls in the suborder Suiformes, family Suidae. Domestic swine (*Sus scrofa domesticus*) are descended from the European wild boar with some input from the smaller *Sus indica* from China. The adjective "porcine" is derived from the Latin *porcinus*, from porcus, a hog. Reflecting its omnivorous diet, the swine's digestive tract is somewhat simpler than those of ruminating animals.

The chicken or domestic fowl (*Gallus gallus domesticus*) is classified with other comb-bearing gallinaceous birds in the order Galliformes. Descended from the Red Junglefowl of southeast Asia, the chicken is in the family Phasianidae.

## GENERAL TERMINOLOGY

With some exceptions, particularly for most muscles wherein traditional Latin names are used, the terminology in this *Atlas* conforms to English translations of Latin terms in the *Nomina Anatomica Veterinaria (N.A.V.)*, 3rd ed., 1983. There are some departures from N.A.V., however. For example, according to N.A.V., the hoof includes the underlying corium (dermis) with the horny epidermis, whereas in common usage hoof refers only to the horny epidermal structure. In compliance with the intent of N.A.V., nomenclature will be consistent for all species. Common terms and meat-packing terms are used on some plates. Abbreviations for organs in this *Atlas* include: a, artery; b, bone; j, joint; lig., ligament; ln, lymph node; m, muscle; n, nerve; v, vein. Double letters indicate the plural form of these words (e.g., aa, arteries). Positional and directional terms, body planes, and the extent of body cavities are used to indicate the location of parts of the body and functional changes in position. The extent of diseased regions is defined using this anatomic terminology.

## POSITIONAL AND DIRECTIONAL TERMS

The following terms are illustrated on the accompanying drawing of a horse. **Dorsal** and **ventral** are opposite terms indicating relative locations toward the back (L., dorsum) or belly (L., venter). Above the knee (carpus) and hock (tarsus) and from the belly to the back, a structure located closer to the cranium (skull case) is **cranial** to another structure, and a structure located toward the tail (L., cauda) is **caudal** to another. On the head, the term **rostral** indicates a structure closer to the nose (L., rostrum).

Proximal indicates a location toward the attached end of a limb; **distal** indicates a location toward the free end of a limb, that is, further from the trunk. Distal to and including the carpus, **dorsal** replaces cranial; **palmar** replaces caudal. Distal to and including the hock, dorsal replaces cranial, but **plantar** replaces caudal.

On a frontal view of the distal end of a limb, notice that an **axial** structure is located toward the axis. An **abaxial** structure is located away from it.

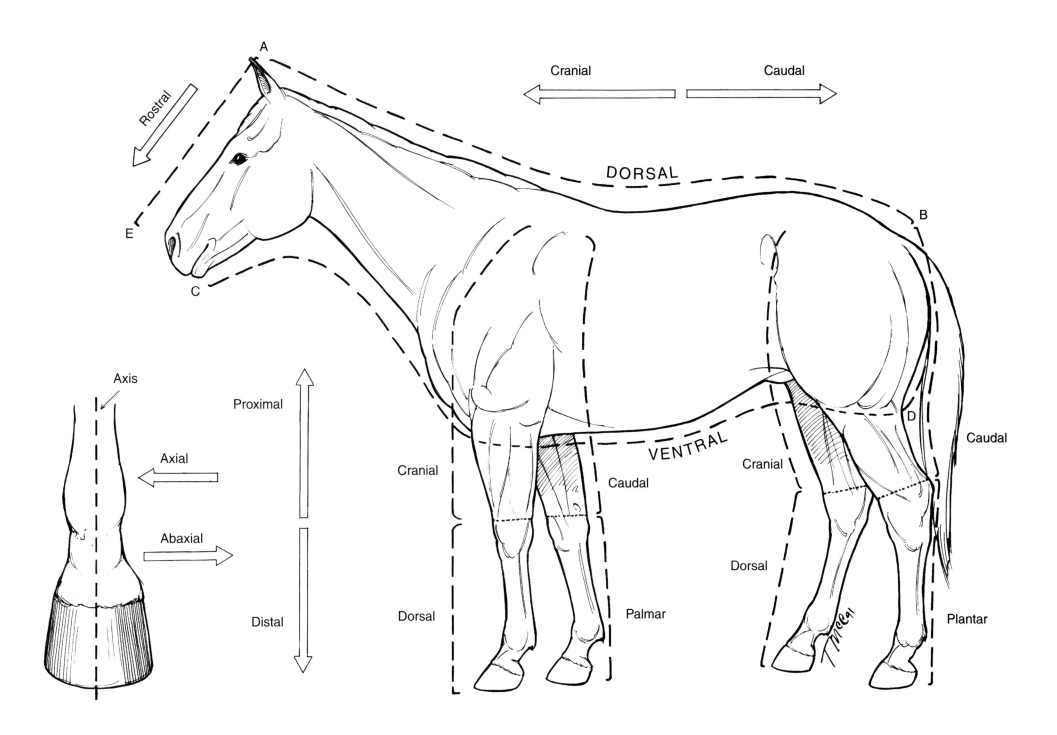

Cranial

Caudal

Rostral

A

DORSAL

B

E

C

Axis

Proximal

VENTRAL

Cranial

Caudal

D

Caudal

Axial

Cranial

Dorsal

Abaxial

Palmar

Plantar

Distal

## BODY PLANES

Drawings of a horse are used to illustrate body planes. The **median plane** (L., medius, middle) divides the animal body into right and left halves. A **sagittal plane** (L., sagitta, arrow) is any plane parallel to the median plane. **Medial** and **lateral** (L., latus, side) are directional terms relative to the median plane. Medial structures are located closer to the median plane. Lateral structures lie away from the median plane, that is, toward the side. A **transverse plane** passes through the head, trunk, or limb perpendicular to the part's long axis. A **dorsal plane** (also called a **frontal plane**) is a longitudinal plane that passes through the body parallel to its dorsal surface at right angles to the median plane.

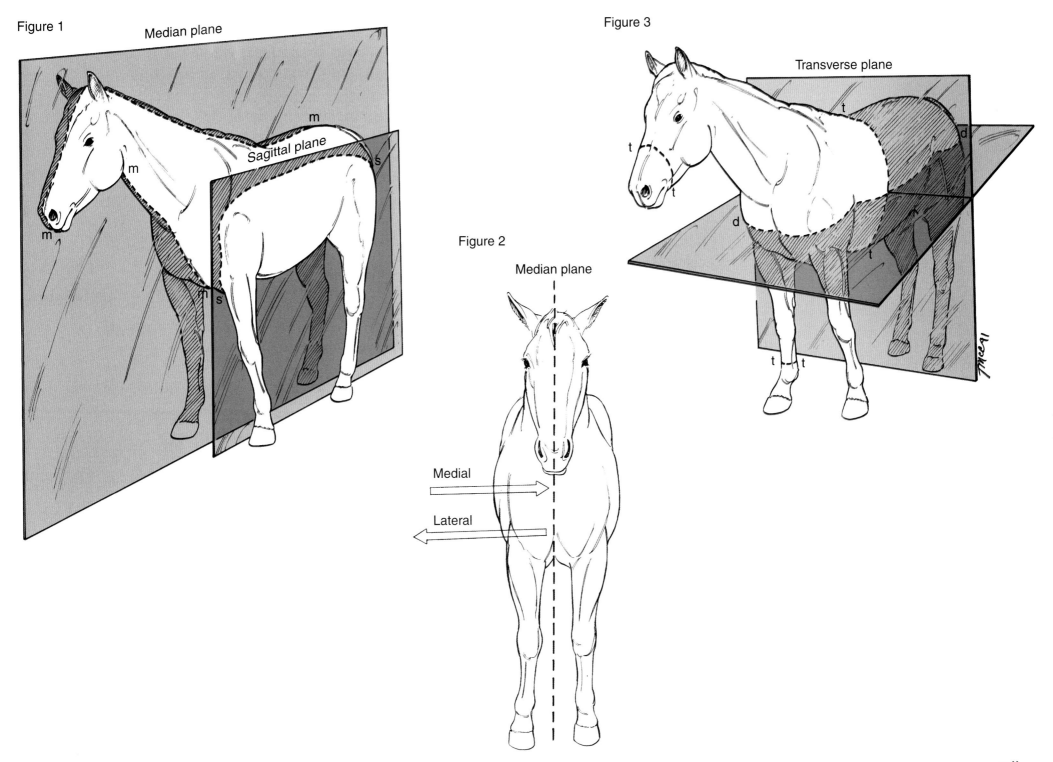

Figure 1

Median plane

m

Sagittal plane

m

s

m

m

s'

Figure 2

Median plane

Medial

Lateral

Figure 3

Transverse plane

t

t

d

t

d

t

t

t

## BODY CAVITIES AND MEMBRANES

A diagrammatic drawing of a mare's trunk illustrates the **thoracic, abdominal,** and **pelvic cavities** and the serous membranes—**peritoneum, pleura,** and **pericardium**—that line the cavities and suspend organs.

The peritoneum consists of three continuous parts. The **parietal peritoneum** (L., paries, wall) lines the abdominal cavity and the cranial part of the pelvic cavity. **Connecting peritoneum** reflects from the parietal peritoneum and suspends organs in a double fold containing vessels and nerves as it extends to an organ. The connecting peritoneum is indicated by mes- (G., mesos, middle) plus the Latin or Greek name of the organ. An example is mesentery: mes- plus G., enteron, small intestine. Peritoneal ligaments suspend and support—e.g., the falciform ligament of the liver. **Visceral peritoneum** is continuous with connecting peritoneum, encircling a viscus (Latin for a large, internal organ; plural, **viscera**).

The musculomembranous **diaphragm** is covered with peritoneum on its abdominal surface and pleura on its thoracic surface.

The **pleurae** are two continuous serous membranes, each forming a pleural sac. The **parietal pleura** lines each half of the thoracic cavity. **Mediastinal pleura** is connecting pleura on each side enclosing the **mediastinum**, a space containing the heart, esophagus, trachea, blood vessels, lymph nodes and ducts, thymus, nerves, and adipose tissue. **Visceral pleura** covers each lung.

The **pericardium** is the heart sac. **Visceral pericardium** (also called epicardium) covers the heart and reflects around the base of the heart and great vessels to become continuous with the **parietal pericardium**.

The serous cavities—**peritoneal cavity, pleural cavity,** and **pericardial cavity**—are potential spaces between parietal and visceral membranes containing lubricating serous fluids named for each cavity.

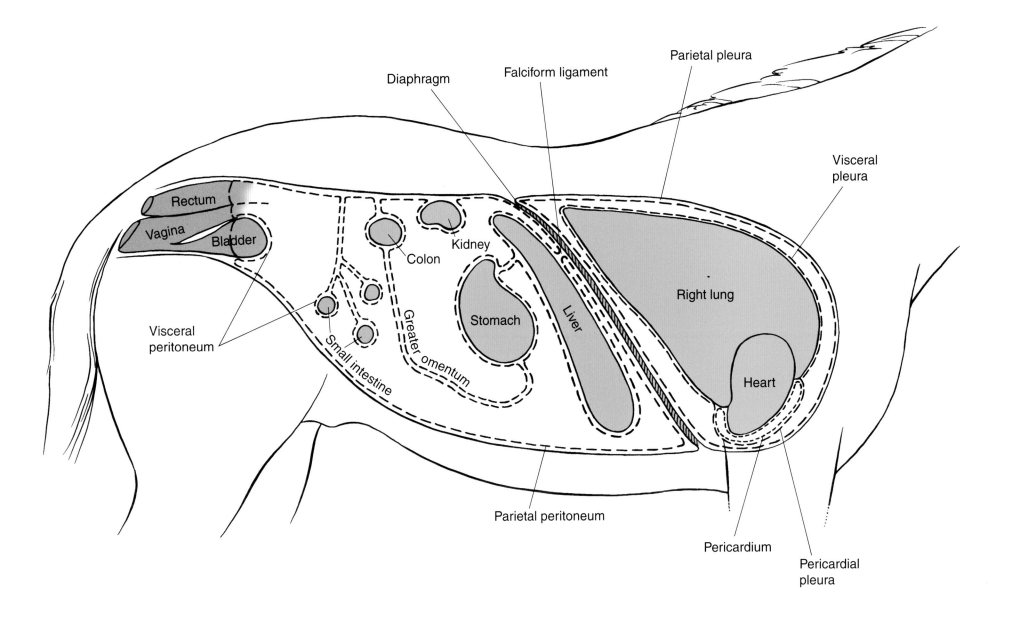

Diaphragm

Falciform ligament

Parietal pleura

Visceral pleura

Rectum

Vagina

Bladder

Colon

Kidney

Right lung

Visceral peritoneum

Stomach

Liver

Small intestine

Greater omentum

Heart

Parietal peritoneum

Pericardium

Pericardial pleura

# SECTION 1   THE HORSE *(Equus caballus)*

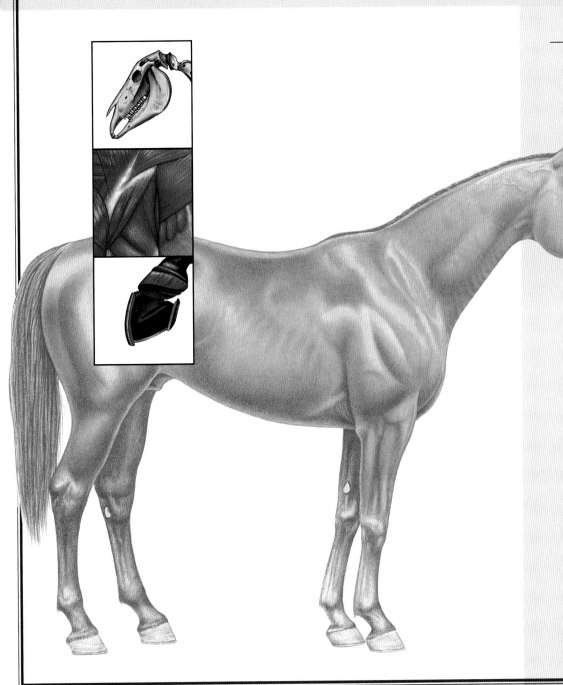

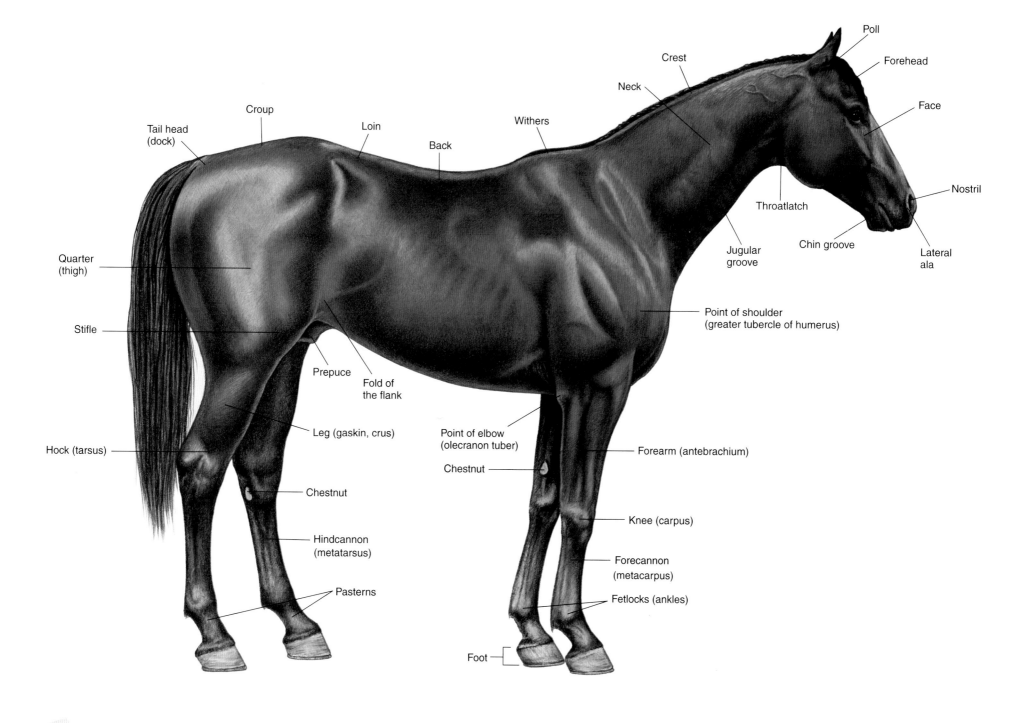

Poll

Crest

Neck

Forehead

Face

Withers

Nostril

Croup

Loin

Throatlatch

Tail head
(dock)

Back

Chin groove

Lateral
ala

Jugular
groove

Quarter
(thigh)

Point of shoulder
(greater tubercle of humerus)

Stifle

Prepuce

Fold of
the flank

Leg (gaskin, crus)

Point of elbow
(olecranon tuber)

Forearm (antebrachium)

Hock (tarsus)

Chestnut

Chestnut

Knee (carpus)

Hindcannon
(metatarsus)

Forecannon
(metacarpus)

Pasterns

Fetlocks (ankles)

Foot

2

**PLATE 1.1**   Right lateral view of a stallion.

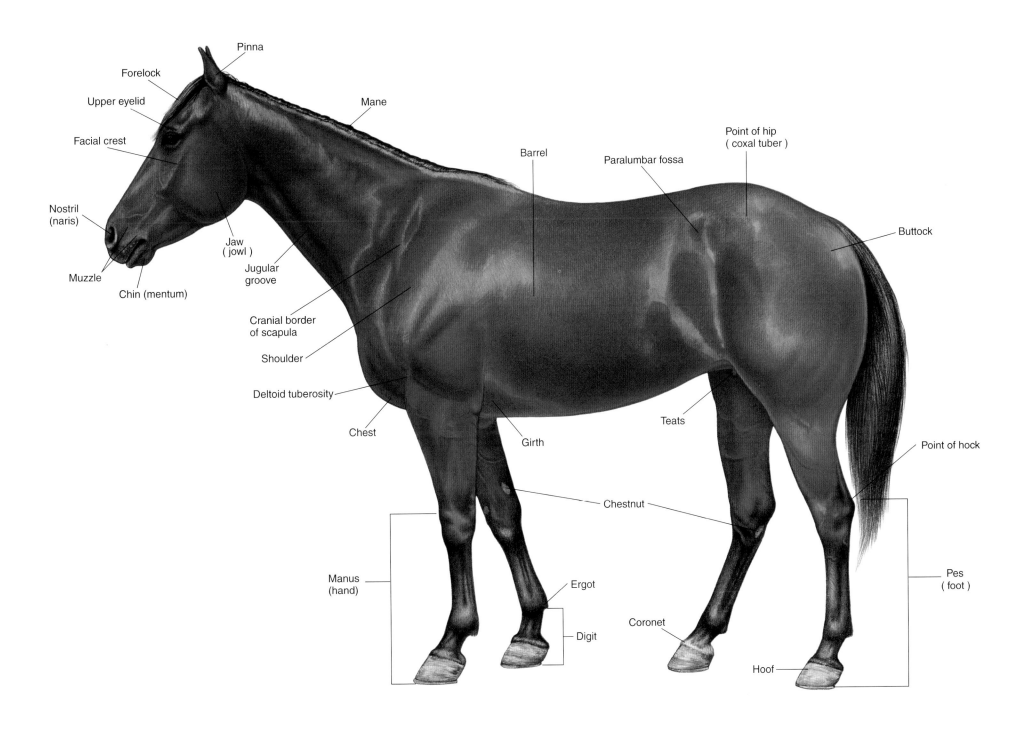

Pinna

Forelock

Upper eyelid

Facial crest

Mane

Barrel

Point of hip
( coxal tuber )

Paralumbar fossa

Nostril
(naris)

Buttock

Jaw
( jowl )

Muzzle

Jugular
groove

Chin (mentum)

Cranial border
of scapula

Shoulder

Deltoid tuberosity

Teats

Chest

Girth

Point of hock

Chestnut

Manus
(hand)

Ergot

Pes
( foot )

Coronet

Digit

Hoof

**PLATE 1.2**   Left lateral view of a mare.

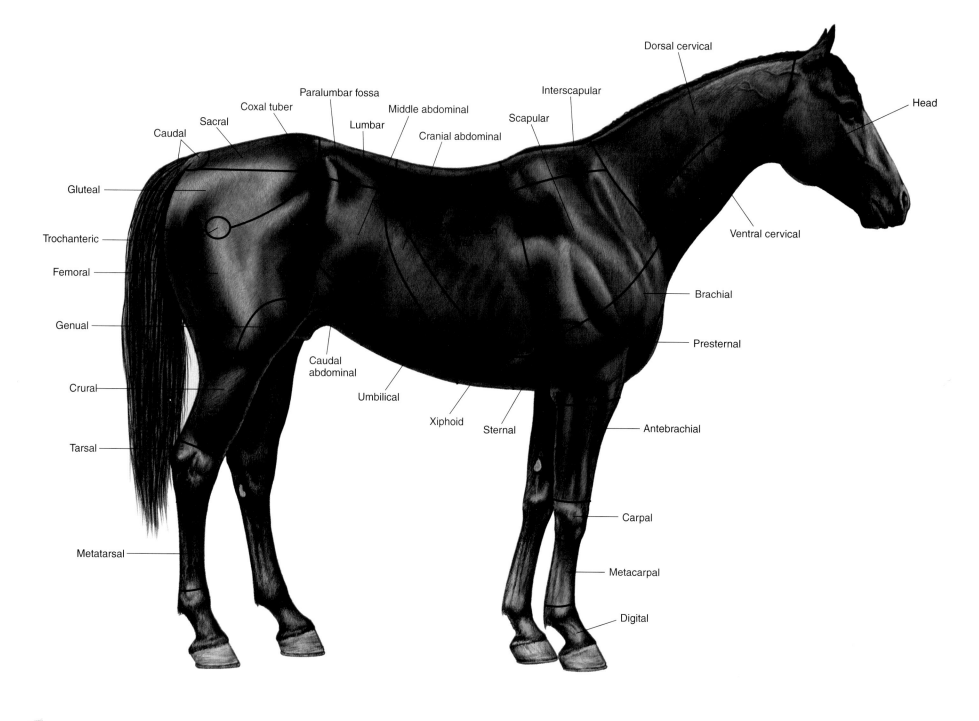

Dorsal cervical

Interscapular

Head

Paralumbar fossa

Coxal tuber

Middle abdominal

Scapular

Lumbar

Cranial abdominal

Sacral

Caudal

Gluteal

Ventral cervical

Trochanteric

Brachial

Femoral

Presternal

Genual

Caudal abdominal

Crural

Umbilical

Antebrachial

Xiphoid

Sternal

Tarsal

Carpal

Metatarsal

Metacarpal

Digital

4

**PLATE 1.3**   Body regions of the horse.  Right lateral view.

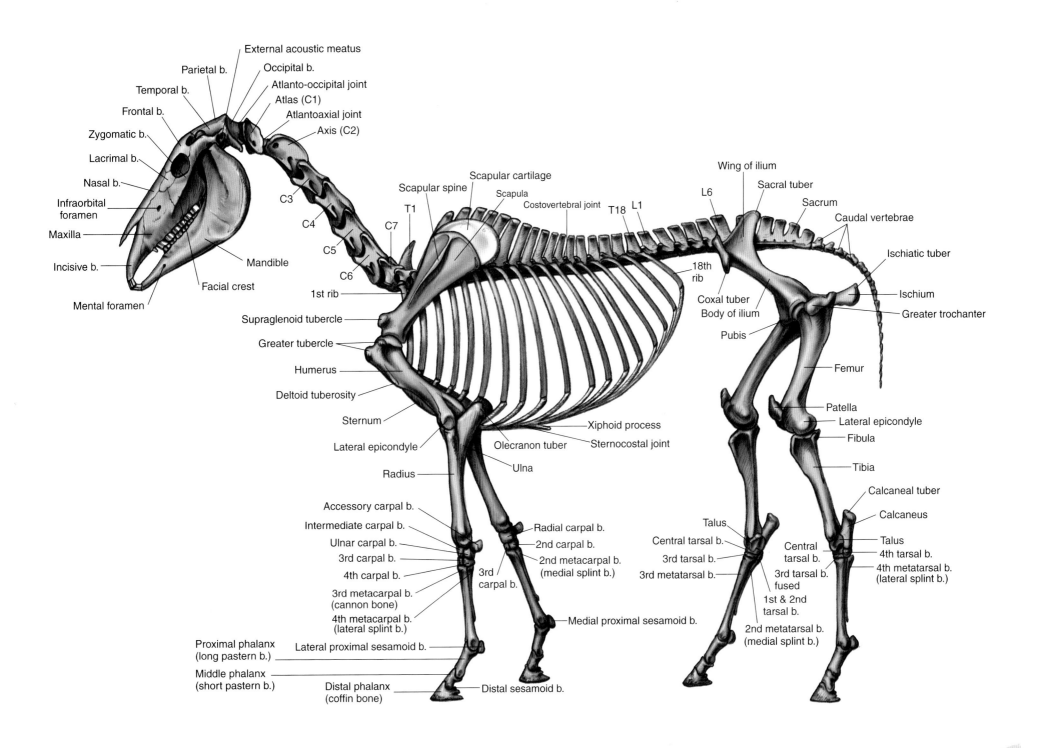

**PLATE 1.4**  Skeleton of the horse.  Left lateral view. C = cervical vertebra,
T = thoracic vertebra, L = lumbar vertebra , b = bone

5

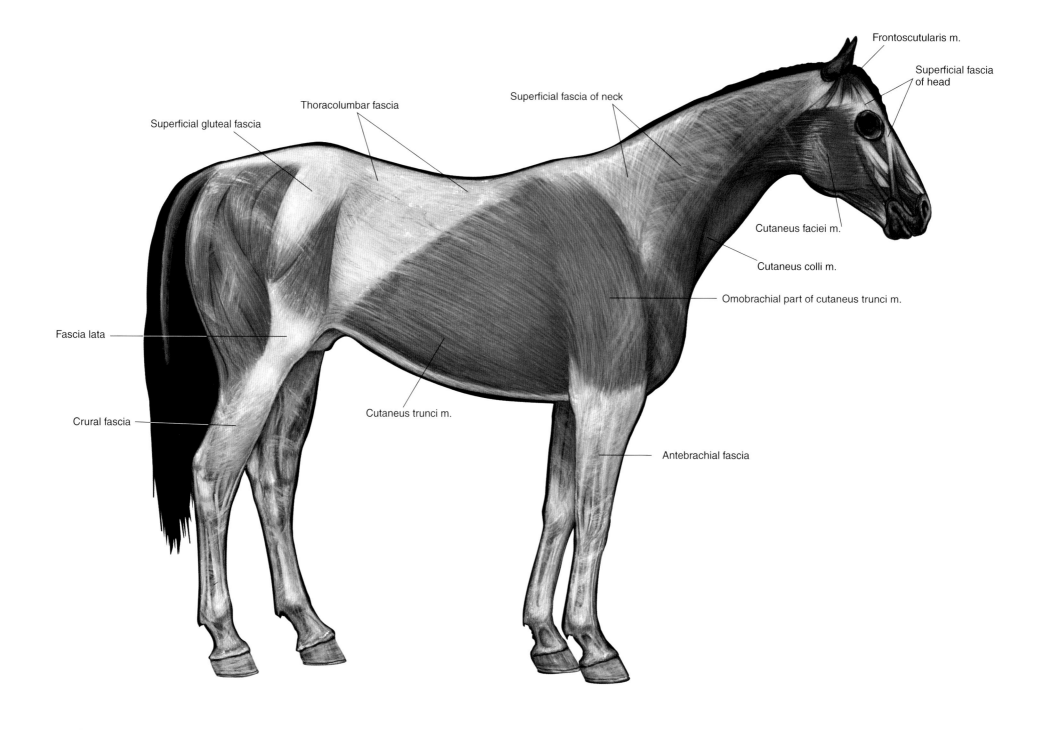

Frontoscutularis m.

Superficial fascia of head

Superficial fascia of neck

Thoracolumbar fascia

Superficial gluteal fascia

Cutaneus faciei m.

Cutaneus colli m.

Omobrachial part of cutaneus trunci m.

Fascia lata

Crural fascia

Cutaneus trunci m.

Antebrachial fascia

**6**

**PLATE 1.5** Cutaneous muscles and major fasciae of the stallion. Right lateral view. m = muscle

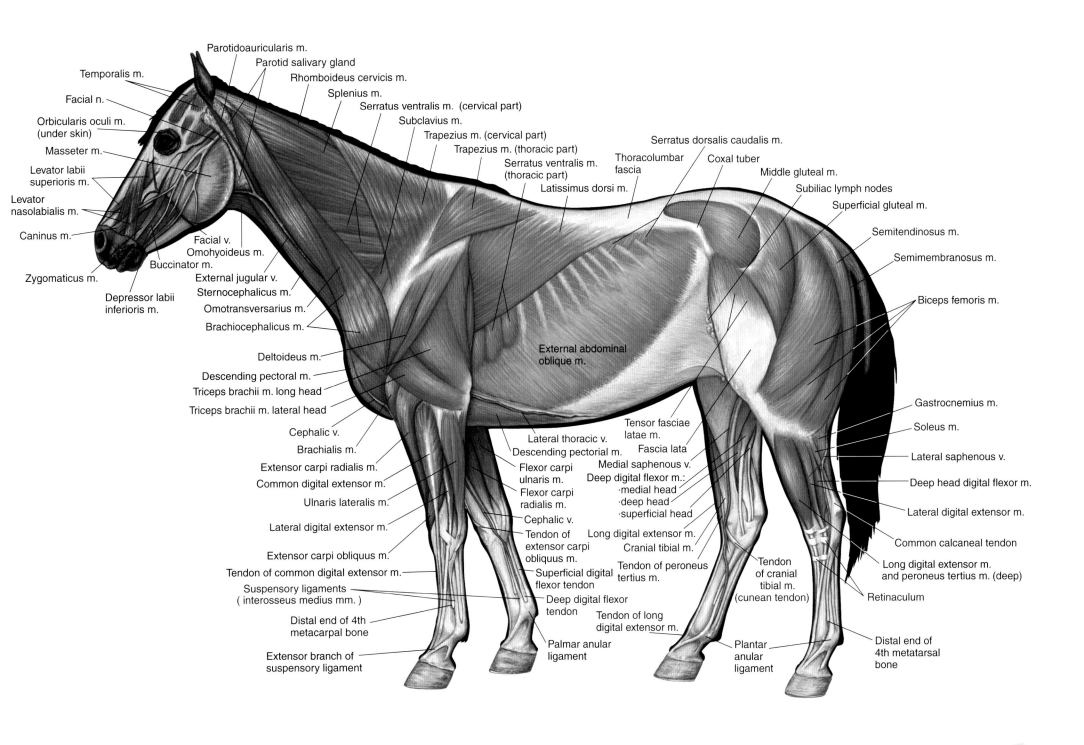

Parotidoauricularis m.
Temporalis m.
Facial n.
Orbicularis oculi m. (under skin)
Masseter m.
Levator labii superioris m.
Levator nasolabialis m.
Caninus m.
Zygomaticus m.
Depressor labii inferioris m.
Buccinator m.
Parotid salivary gland
Rhomboideus cervicis m.
Splenius m.
Serratus ventralis m. (cervical part)
Subclavius m.
Trapezius m. (cervical part)
Trapezius m. (thoracic part)
Serratus ventralis m. (thoracic part)
Latissimus dorsi m.
Facial v.
Omohyoideus m.
External jugular v.
Sternocephalicus m.
Omotransversarius m.
Brachiocephalicus m.
Deltoideus m.
Descending pectoral m.
Triceps brachii m. long head
Triceps brachii m. lateral head
Cephalic v.
Brachialis m.
Extensor carpi radialis m.
Common digital extensor m.
Ulnaris lateralis m.
Lateral digital extensor m.
Extensor carpi obliquus m.
Tendon of common digital extensor m.
Suspensory ligaments ( interosseus medius mm. )
Distal end of 4th metacarpal bone
Extensor branch of suspensory ligament

Serratus dorsalis caudalis m.
Thoracolumbar fascia
Coxal tuber
Middle gluteal m.
Subiliac lymph nodes
Superficial gluteal m.
Semitendinosus m.
Semimembranosus m.
Biceps femoris m.

External abdominal oblique m.

Tensor fasciae latae m.
Lateral thoracic v.
Descending pectoral m.
Fascia lata
Flexor carpi ulnaris m.
Medial saphenous v.
Flexor carpi radialis m.
Deep digital flexor m.:
·medial head
·deep head
·superficial head
Cephalic v.
Tendon of extensor carpi obliquus m.
Long digital extensor m.
Cranial tibial m.
Superficial digital flexor tendon
Tendon of peroneus tertius m.
Deep digital flexor tendon
Tendon of long digital extensor m.
Palmar anular ligament
Tendon of cranial tibial m. (cunean tendon)
Plantar anular ligament

Gastrocnemius m.
Soleus m.
Lateral saphenous v.
Deep head digital flexor m.
Lateral digital extensor m.
Common calcaneal tendon
Long digital extensor m. and peroneus tertius m. (deep)
Retinaculum
Distal end of 4th metatarsal bone

7

**PLATE 1.6** Superficial muscles and veins of the mare. Left lateral view.
m = muscle, n = nerve, v = vein

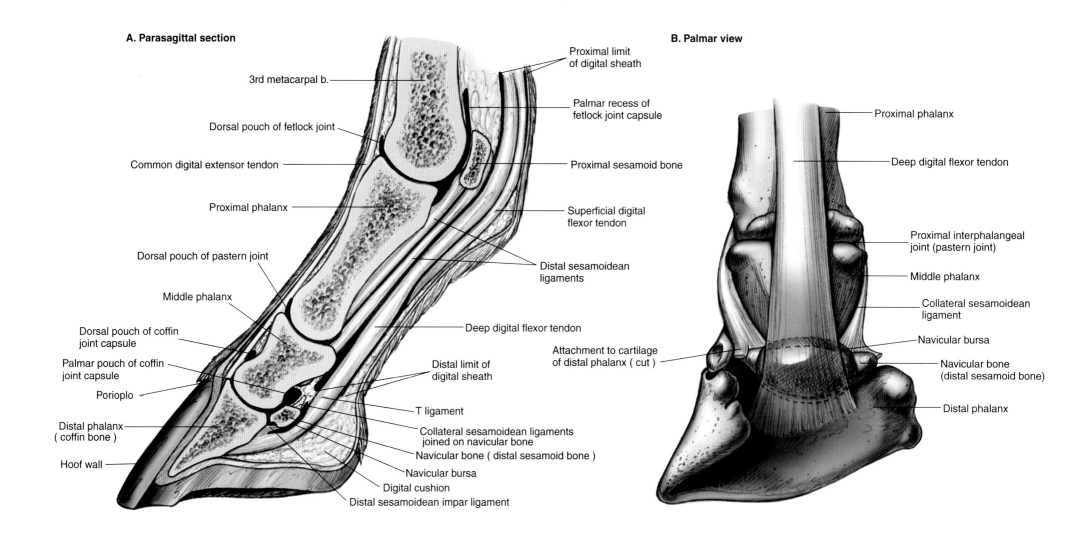

**A. Parasagittal section**

3rd metacarpal b.

Dorsal pouch of fetlock joint

Common digital extensor tendon

Proximal phalanx

Dorsal pouch of pastern joint

Middle phalanx

Dorsal pouch of coffin joint capsule

Palmar pouch of coffin joint capsule

Porioplo

Distal phalanx ( coffin bone )

Hoof wall

Proximal limit of digital sheath

Palmar recess of fetlock joint capsule

Proximal sesamoid bone

Superficial digital flexor tendon

Distal sesamoidean ligaments

Deep digital flexor tendon

Distal limit of digital sheath

T ligament

Collateral sesamoidean ligaments joined on navicular bone

Navicular bone ( distal sesamoid bone )

Navicular bursa

Digital cushion

Distal sesamoidean impar ligament

**B. Palmar view**

Proximal phalanx

Deep digital flexor tendon

Proximal interphalangeal joint (pastern joint)

Middle phalanx

Collateral sesamoidean ligament

Navicular bursa

Navicular bone (distal sesamoid bone)

Distal phalanx

Attachment to cartilage of distal phalanx ( cut )

**PLATE 1.7** **A.** Parasagittal section of the equine digit. **B.** Palmar (plantar) view of major structures of the equine digit. Navicular bursa obscures joining of collateral sesamoidean ligaments on the navicular bone. b = bone

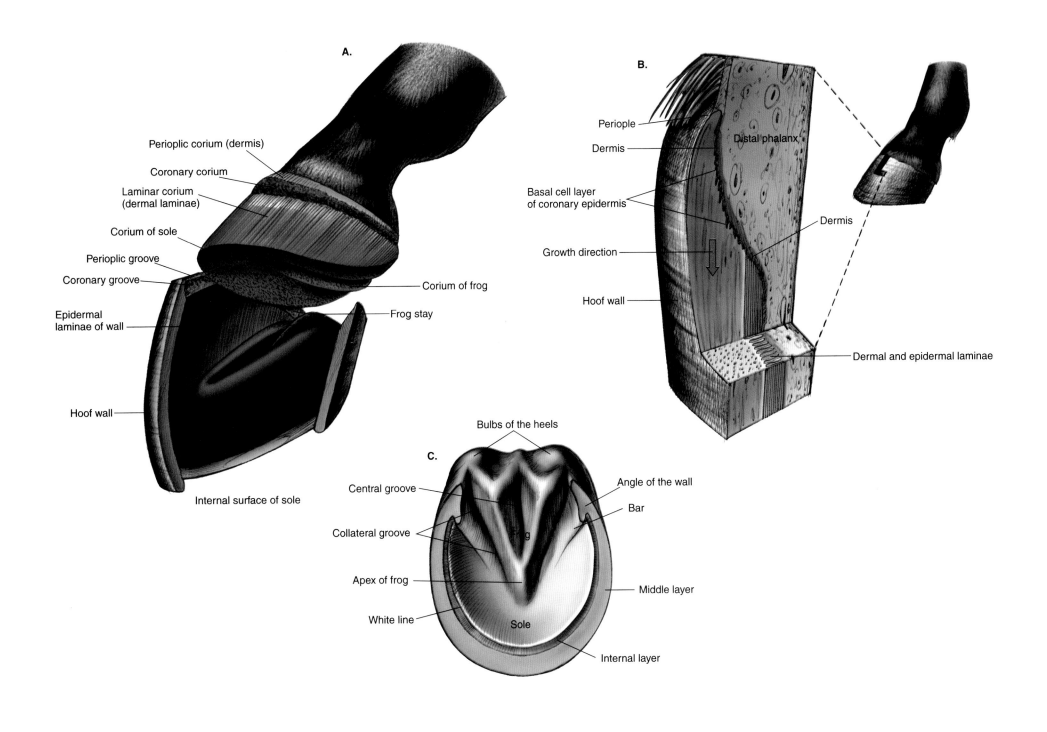

**A.**

Perioplic corium (dermis)

Coronary corium

Laminar corium (dermal laminae)

Corium of sole

Perioplic groove

Coronary groove

Epidermal laminae of wall

Hoof wall

Internal surface of sole

Corium of frog

Frog stay

**B.**

Periople

Dermis

Basal cell layer of coronary epidermis

Growth direction

Hoof wall

Distal phalanx

Dermis

Dermal and epidermal laminae

**C.**

Bulbs of the heels

Central groove

Collateral groove

Apex of frog

White line

Angle of the wall

Bar

Frog

Sole

Middle layer

Internal layer

**PLATE 1.8** Relations of the hoof. **A.** Separation of the hoof to show its relations to regions of the corium. **B.** Three-dimensional dissection to show relations of the hoof wall, coronary and laminar corium, and distal phalanx. **C.** Solar surface of the hoof.

9

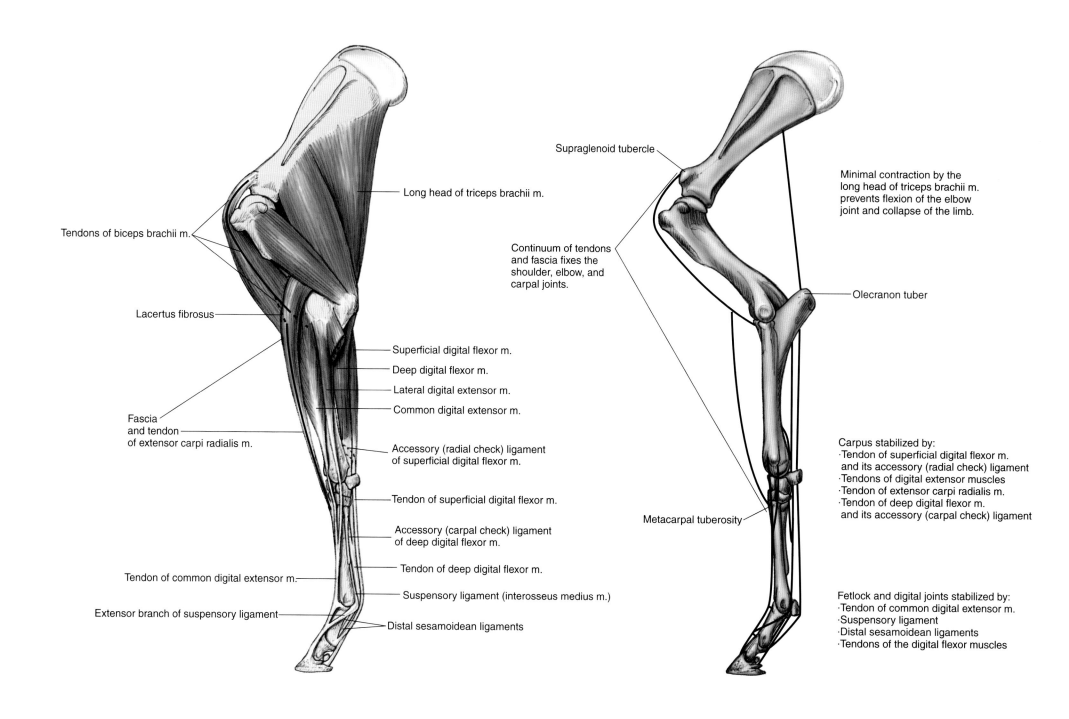

Supraglenoid tubercle

Long head of triceps brachii m.

Tendons of biceps brachii m.

Continuum of tendons
and fascia fixes the
shoulder, elbow, and
carpal joints.

Minimal contraction by the
long head of triceps brachii m.
prevents flexion of the elbow
joint and collapse of the limb.

Lacertus fibrosus

Olecranon tuber

Superficial digital flexor m.

Deep digital flexor m.

Lateral digital extensor m.

Common digital extensor m.

Fascia
and tendon
of extensor carpi radialis m.

Accessory (radial check) ligament
of superficial digital flexor m.

Carpus stabilized by:
·Tendon of superficial digital flexor m.
 and its accessory (radial check) ligament
·Tendons of digital extensor muscles
·Tendon of extensor carpi radialis m.
·Tendon of deep digital flexor m.
 and its accessory (carpal check) ligament

Tendon of superficial digital flexor m.

Accessory (carpal check) ligament
of deep digital flexor m.

Metacarpal tuberosity

Tendon of deep digital flexor m.

Tendon of common digital extensor m.

Suspensory ligament (interosseus medius m.)

Extensor branch of suspensory ligament

Distal sesamoidean ligaments

Fetlock and digital joints stabilized by:
·Tendon of common digital extensor m.
·Suspensory ligament
·Distal sesamoidean ligaments
·Tendons of the digital flexor muscles

10

**PLATE 1.9**   Stay apparatus of the equine forelimb.  The continuum of tendons and ligaments with
minimal muscular activity stabilizes joints of the forelimb in the standing position. m = muscle

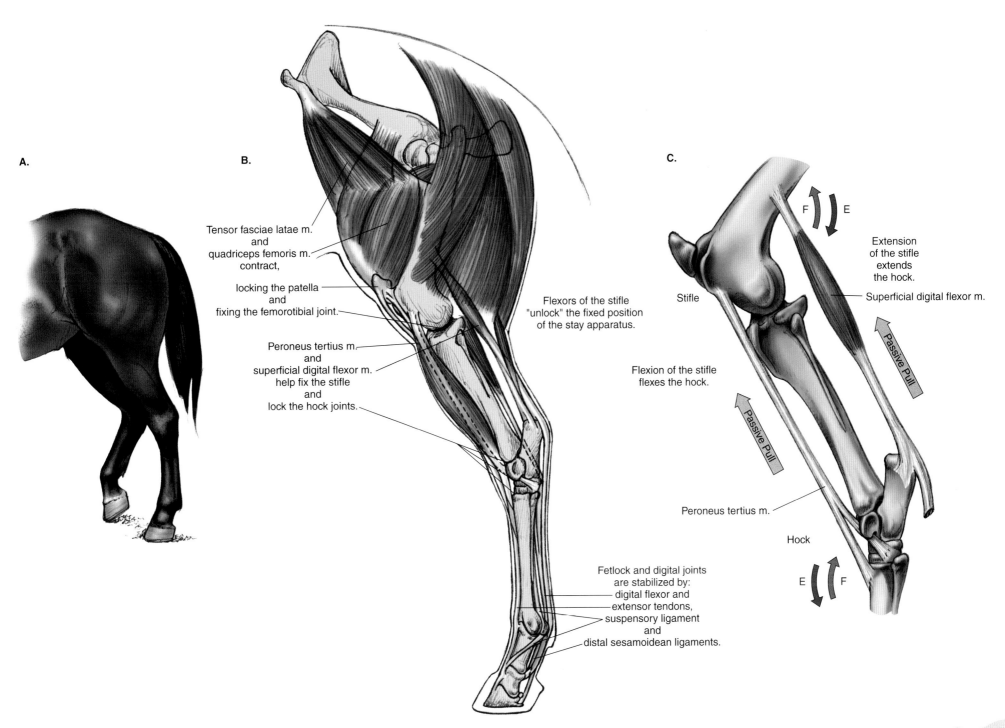

**A.**

**B.**

Tensor fasciae latae m.
and
quadriceps femoris m.
contract,

locking the patella
and
fixing the femorotibial joint.

Peroneus tertius m.
and
superficial digital flexor m.
help fix the stifle
and
lock the hock joints.

Flexors of the stifle
"unlock" the fixed position
of the stay apparatus.

Fetlock and digital joints
are stabilized by:
digital flexor and
extensor tendons,
suspensory ligament
and
distal sesamoidean ligaments.

**C.**

F   E

Extension
of the stifle
extends
the hock.

Stifle

Superficial digital flexor m.

Passive Pull

Flexion of the stifle
flexes the hock.

Passive Pull

Peroneus tertius m.

Hock

E   F

**PLATE 1.10**   Stay apparatus and reciprocal apparatus of the hindlimb.  **A.** One hindlimb partly
flexed with its toe on the ground, and the foot of the opposite limb fixed with minimal
muscular activity by the stay apparatus.  **B.** Stay apparatus of the
hindlimb.  **C.** The reciprocal apparatus. m = muscle

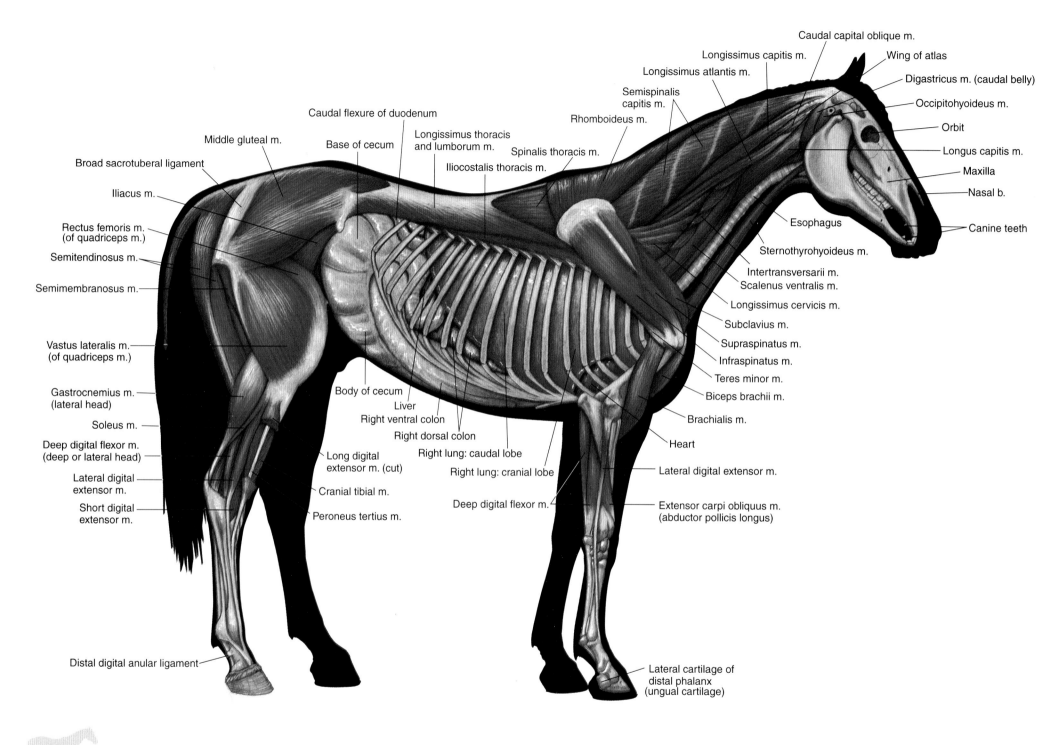

Caudal capital oblique m.

Longissimus capitis m.

Wing of atlas

Longissimus atlantis m.

Digastricus m. (caudal belly)

Semispinalis capitis m.

Occipitohyoideus m.

Rhomboideus m.

Orbit

Caudal flexure of duodenum

Middle gluteal m.

Longissimus thoracis and lumborum m.

Longus capitis m.

Base of cecum

Spinalis thoracis m.

Broad sacrotuberal ligament

Maxilla

Iliocostalis thoracis m.

Nasal b.

Iliacus m.

Esophagus

Rectus femoris m. (of quadriceps m.)

Canine teeth

Sternothyrohyoideus m.

Semitendinosus m.

Intertransversarii m.

Semimembranosus m.

Scalenus ventralis m.

Longissimus cervicis m.

Subclavius m.

Vastus lateralis m. (of quadriceps m.)

Supraspinatus m.

Infraspinatus m.

Teres minor m.

Gastrocnemius m. (lateral head)

Biceps brachii m.

Body of cecum

Brachialis m.

Soleus m.

Liver

Deep digital flexor m. (deep or lateral head)

Right ventral colon

Heart

Right dorsal colon

Lateral digital extensor m.

Long digital extensor m. (cut)

Right lung: caudal lobe

Lateral digital extensor m.

Cranial tibial m.

Right lung: cranial lobe

Short digital extensor m.

Extensor carpi obliquus m. (abductor pollicis longus)

Peroneus tertius m.

Deep digital flexor m.

Distal digital anular ligament

Lateral cartilage of distal phalanx (ungual cartilage)

**12**

**PLATE 1.11**  Deep muscles and *in situ* viscera of the stallion.
Right lateral view. m = muscle, b = bone

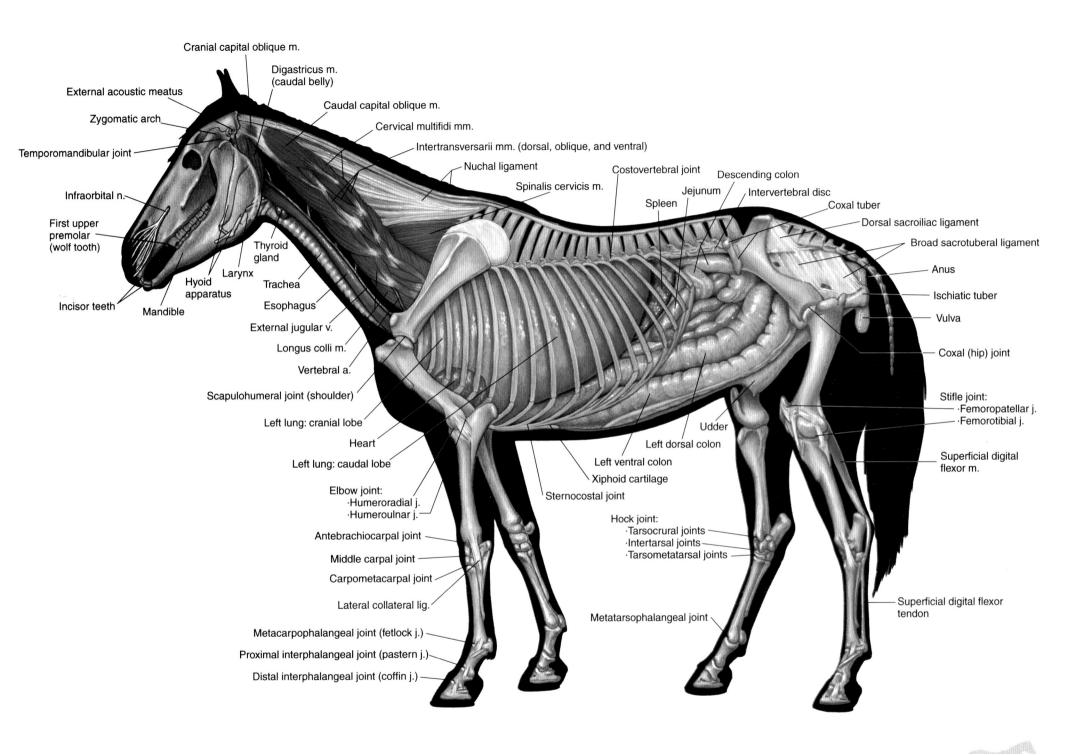

**PLATE 1.12** Deep cervical muscles, major joints, and *in situ* viscera of the mare. Left lateral view.
n = nerve, v = vein, m = muscle, a = artery, j = joint, lig = ligament

13

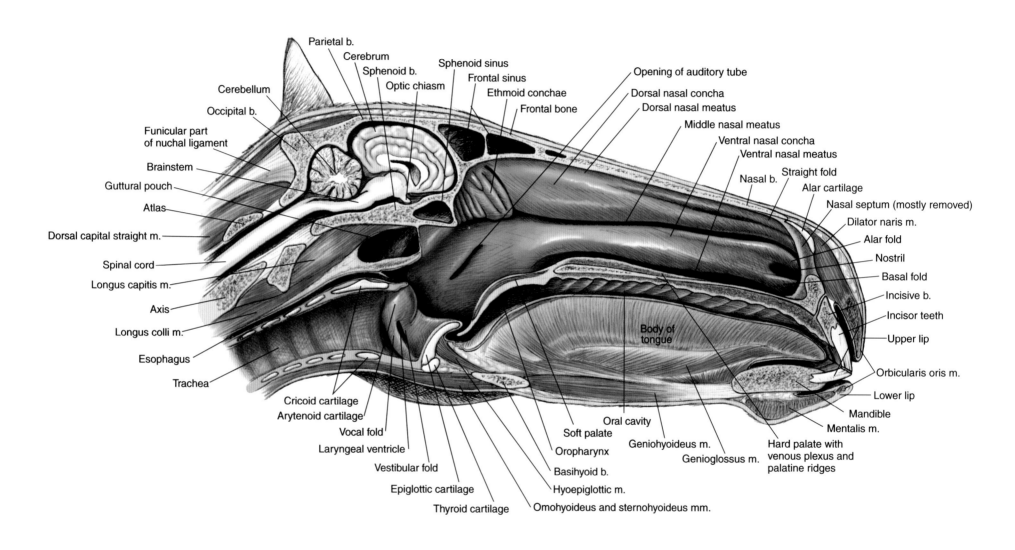

**PLATE 1.13** Median section of the horse's head. Nasal septum mostly removed.
b = bone, m = muscle

Parietal b.
Cerebrum
Sphenoid b.
Optic chiasm
Cerebellum
Occipital b.
Funicular part of nuchal ligament
Brainstem
Guttural pouch
Atlas
Dorsal capital straight m.
Spinal cord
Longus capitis m.
Axis
Longus colli m.
Esophagus
Trachea
Sphenoid sinus
Frontal sinus
Ethmoid conchae
Frontal bone
Opening of auditory tube
Dorsal nasal concha
Dorsal nasal meatus
Middle nasal meatus
Ventral nasal concha
Ventral nasal meatus
Straight fold
Nasal b.
Alar cartilage
Nasal septum (mostly removed)
Dilator naris m.
Alar fold
Nostril
Basal fold
Incisive b.
Incisor teeth
Body of tongue
Upper lip
Orbicularis oris m.
Lower lip
Mandible
Mentalis m.
Hard palate with venous plexus and palatine ridges
Cricoid cartilage
Arytenoid cartilage
Vocal fold
Laryngeal ventricle
Vestibular fold
Epiglottic cartilage
Thyroid cartilage
Oral cavity
Soft palate
Geniohyoideus m.
Oropharynx
Genioglossus m.
Basihyoid b.
Hyoepiglottic m.
Omohyoideus and sternohyoideus mm.

14

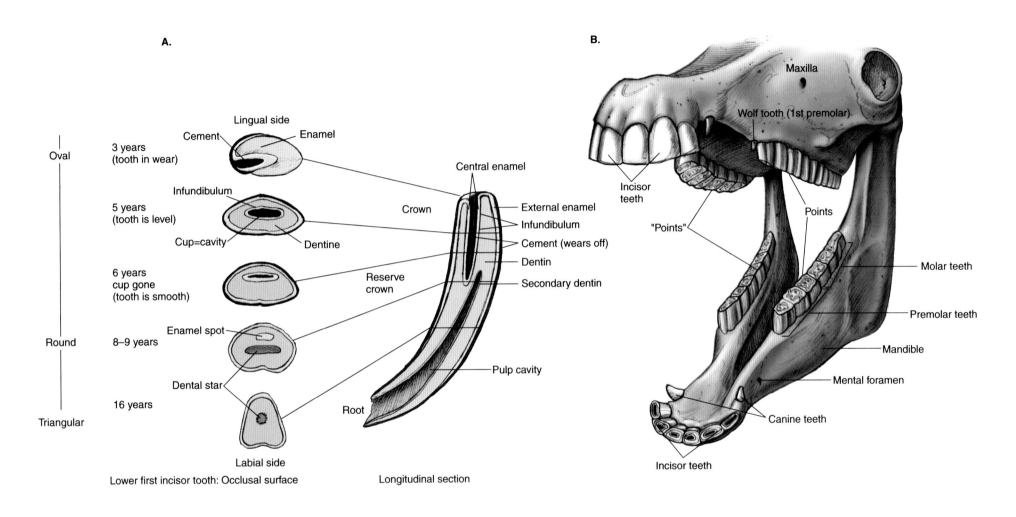

**A.** Oval — Round — Triangular

Lingual side

Cement — Enamel

3 years (tooth in wear)

Infundibulum

5 years (tooth is level)

Cup=cavity — Dentine

6 years cup gone (tooth is smooth)

Enamel spot

8–9 years

Dental star

16 years

Labial side

Lower first incisor tooth: Occlusal surface

Central enamel

Crown

External enamel
Infundibulum
Cement (wears off)
Dentin
Secondary dentin

Reserve crown

Pulp cavity

Root

Longitudinal section

**B.** Maxilla

Wolf tooth (1st premolar)

Incisor teeth

"Points"

Points

Molar teeth

Premolar teeth

Mandible

Mental foramen

Canine teeth

Incisor teeth

**PLATE 1.14   A.** Occlusal (grinding) surfaces of an equine lower first incisor tooth related to continuous eruption and wear. Approximate levels at advancing ages indicated on a longitudinal section. **B.** Complete dentition of the male horse circa 5 years of age.

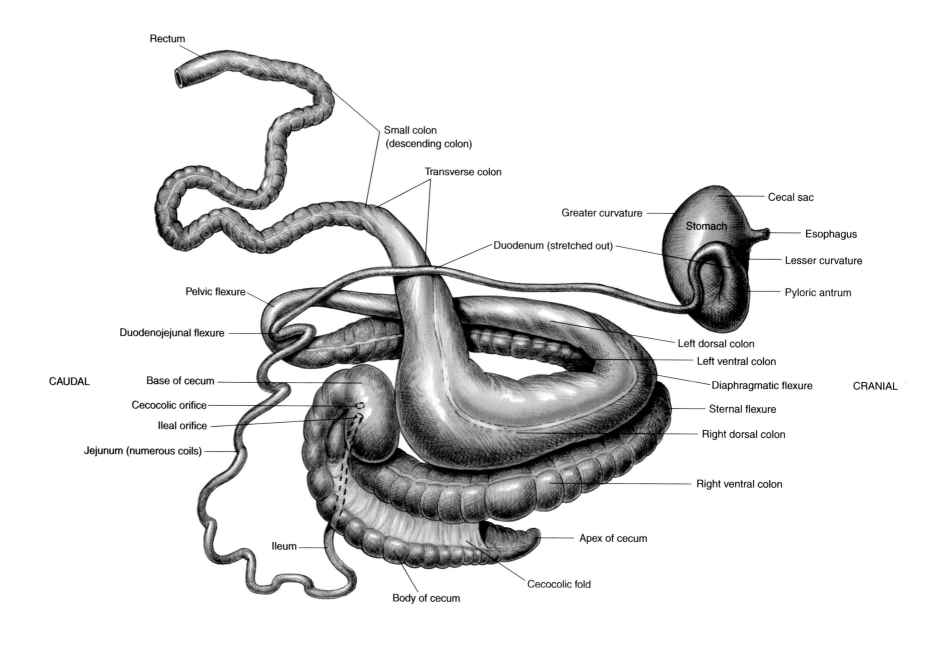

Rectum

Small colon
(descending colon)

Transverse colon

Cecal sac

Greater curvature

Stomach

Esophagus

Lesser curvature

Duodenum (stretched out)

Pyloric antrum

Pelvic flexure

Duodenojejunal flexure

Left dorsal colon

Left ventral colon

CAUDAL

Base of cecum

Diaphragmatic flexure

CRANIAL

Cecocolic orifice

Ileal orifice

Sternal flexure

Right dorsal colon

Jejunum (numerous coils)

Right ventral colon

Apex of cecum

Ileum

Cecocolic fold

Body of cecum

16

**PLATE 1.15**  Isolated stomach and intestines of the horse.

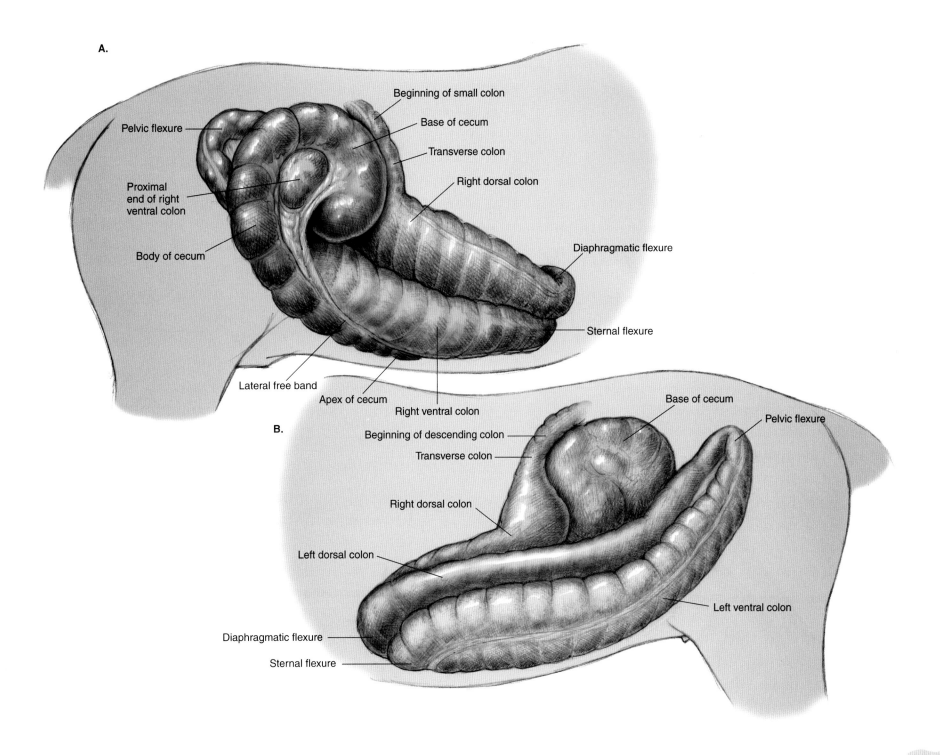

**A.**

Pelvic flexure

Proximal end of right ventral colon

Body of cecum

Lateral free band

Apex of cecum

Beginning of small colon

Base of cecum

Transverse colon

Right dorsal colon

Diaphragmatic flexure

Sternal flexure

Right ventral colon

**B.**

Beginning of descending colon

Transverse colon

Right dorsal colon

Left dorsal colon

Diaphragmatic flexure

Sternal flexure

Base of cecum

Pelvic flexure

Left ventral colon

**PLATE 1.16** Equine cecum, large (ascending) colon, and transverse colon *in situ*.
**A.** Right lateral view. **B.** Left lateral view.

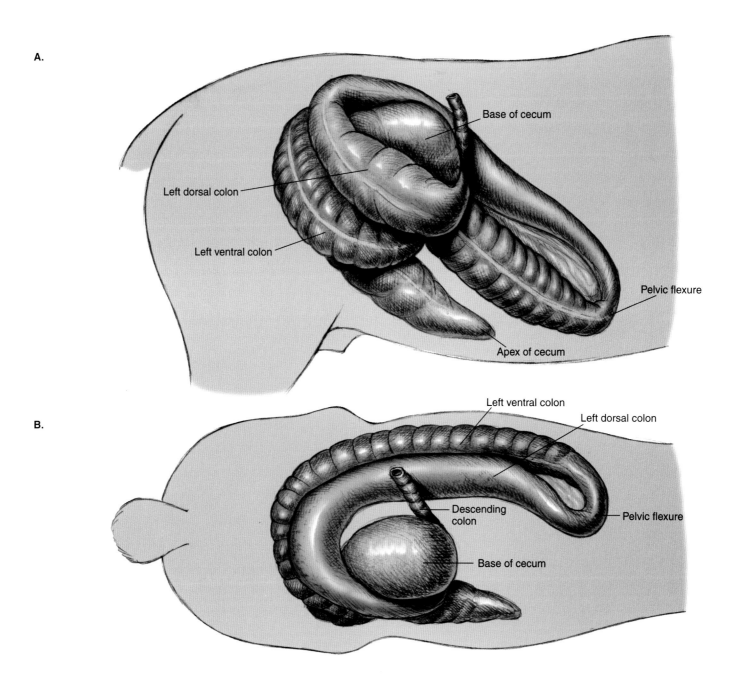

**A.**

Base of cecum

Left dorsal colon

Left ventral colon

Pelvic flexure

Apex of cecum

**B.**

Left ventral colon

Left dorsal colon

Descending colon

Pelvic flexure

Base of cecum

**PLATE 1.17**  Clinical condition: Right dorsal displacement of the large colon.  **A.** Right lateral view.
**B.** Dorsal view.  This displacement is a common cause of colic in adult horses.  Most commonly, the
large colon moves from the left side of the abdomen, courses caudad between the right body wall
and the cecum, and comes to lie again in the left portion of the abdomen with the pelvic flexure
facing toward the diaphragm.  In many cases, the pelvic flexure will not migrate that far
craniad and will instead be located in the caudal aspect of the abdomen on either
side of the body or the median plane.

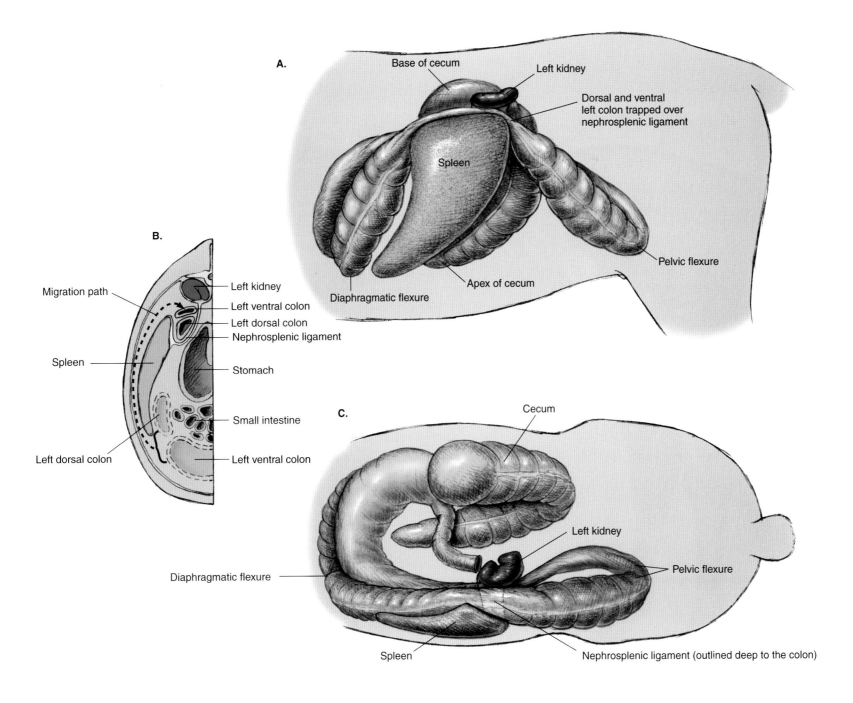

**A.**
Base of cecum
Left kidney
Dorsal and ventral left colon trapped over nephrosplenic ligament
Spleen
Pelvic flexure
Apex of cecum
Diaphragmatic flexure

**B.**
Migration path
Left kidney
Left ventral colon
Left dorsal colon
Nephrosplenic ligament
Spleen
Stomach
Small intestine
Left dorsal colon
Left ventral colon

**C.**
Cecum
Left kidney
Pelvic flexure
Diaphragmatic flexure
Spleen
Nephrosplenic ligament (outlined deep to the colon)

**PLATE 1.18**   Clinical condition: Left dorsal displacement of the large colon.   **A.** Left lateral view. **B.** Cross-section of the left side of the abdomen. Caudocranial view.   **C.** Dorsal view. In this displacement, the left colon moves dorsad and becomes entrapped over the nephrosplenic ligament. The abnormal position of the left colon can often be confirmed by rectal examination, and, many times, left dorsal displacement can be corrected by anesthetizing and rolling the horse to free the entrapment.

19

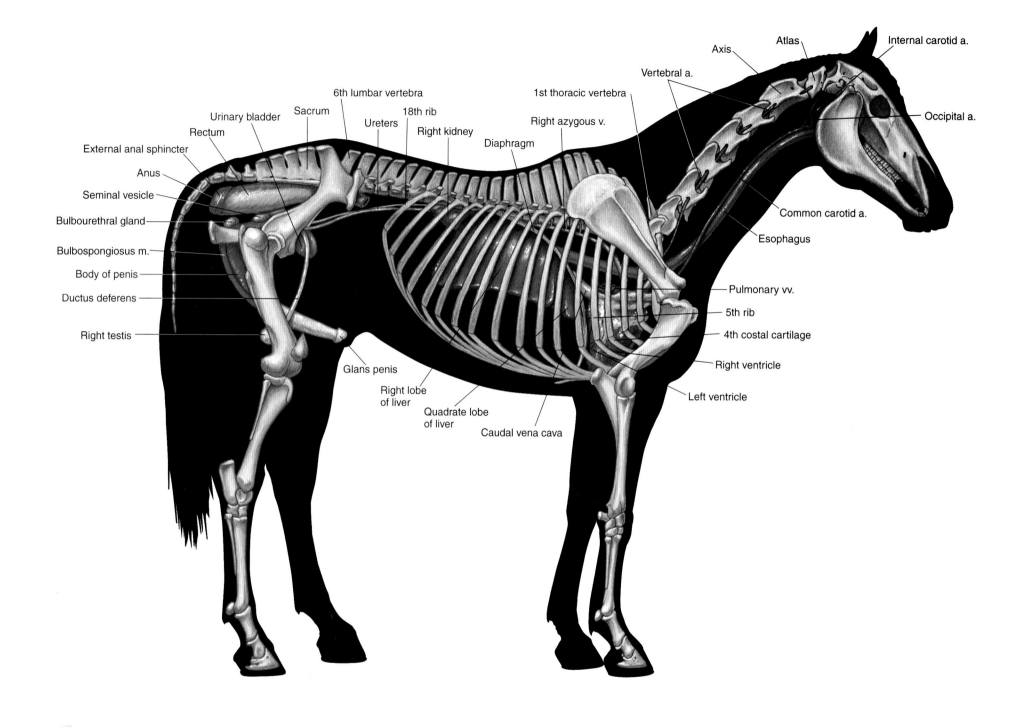

Internal carotid a.

Atlas

Axis

Vertebral a.

1st thoracic vertebra

Right azygous v.

6th lumbar vertebra

Sacrum

Urinary bladder

18th rib

Ureters

Rectum

Right kidney

Diaphragm

External anal sphincter

Anus

Seminal vesicle

Bulbourethral gland

Bulbospongiosus m.

Body of penis

Ductus deferens

Right testis

Occipital a.

Common carotid a.

Esophagus

Pulmonary vv.

5th rib

4th costal cartilage

Right ventricle

Left ventricle

Glans penis

Right lobe
of liver

Quadrate lobe
of liver

Caudal vena cava

**PLATE 1.19**  Reproductive organs, urinary organs, liver, heart, and adjacent major vessels
related to the skeleton of the stallion. Intestines and lungs are removed.
Right lateral view. v = vein, a = artery, m = muscle

20

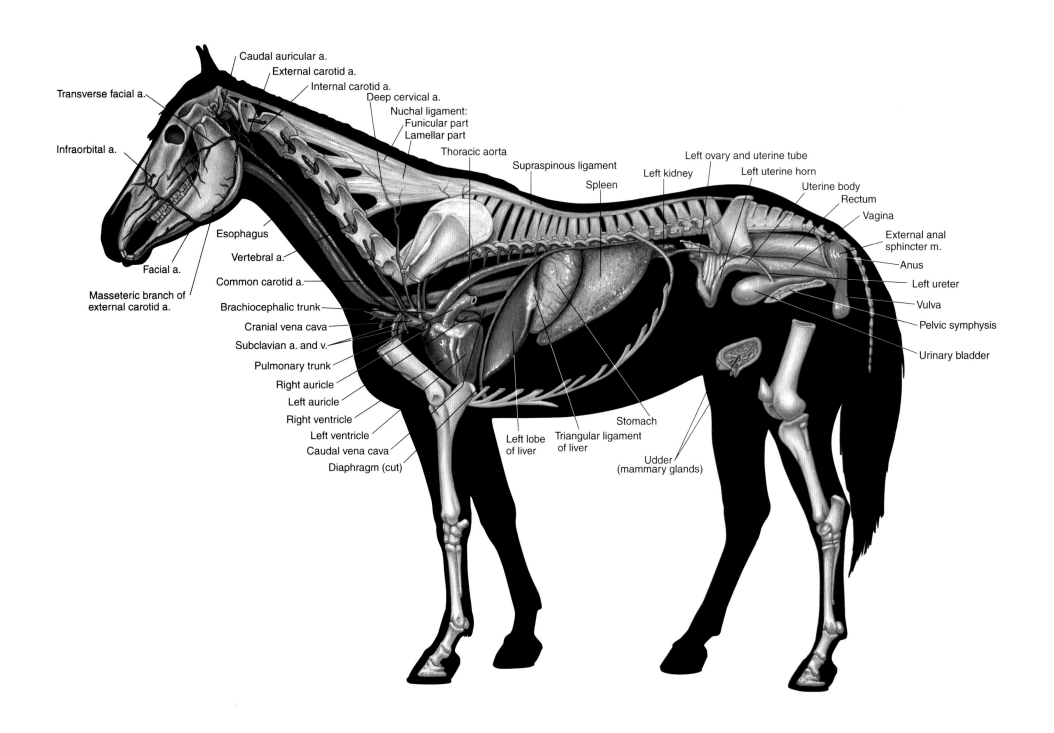

Caudal auricular a.
External carotid a.
Internal carotid a.
Deep cervical a.
Nuchal ligament:
Funicular part
Lamellar part
Thoracic aorta
Supraspinous ligament
Spleen
Left ovary and uterine tube
Left kidney
Left uterine horn
Uterine body
Rectum
Vagina
External anal sphincter m.
Anus
Left ureter
Vulva
Pelvic symphysis
Urinary bladder

Transverse facial a.
Infraorbital a.
Facial a.
Masseteric branch of external carotid a.
Esophagus
Vertebral a.
Common carotid a.
Brachiocephalic trunk
Cranial vena cava
Subclavian a. and v.
Pulmonary trunk
Right auricle
Left auricle
Right ventricle
Left ventricle
Caudal vena cava
Diaphragm (cut)
Left lobe of liver
Triangular ligament of liver
Stomach
Udder (mammary glands)

**PLATE 1.20** Heart and some adjacent major vessels, abdominal and pelvic viscera, and udder (mammary glands) of the mare. Intestines and lungs are removed. Left lateral view. a = artery, v = vein, m = muscle

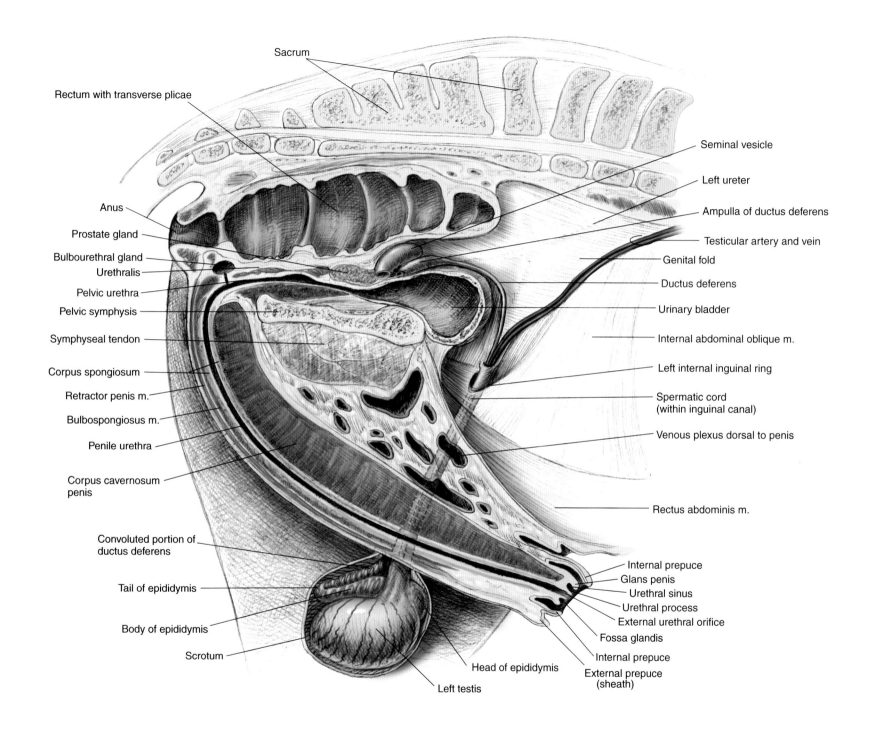

Sacrum

Rectum with transverse plicae

Seminal vesicle

Left ureter

Ampulla of ductus deferens

Anus

Prostate gland

Testicular artery and vein

Bulbourethral gland

Genital fold

Urethralis

Ductus deferens

Pelvic urethra

Urinary bladder

Pelvic symphysis

Internal abdominal oblique m.

Symphyseal tendon

Left internal inguinal ring

Corpus spongiosum

Spermatic cord
(within inguinal canal)

Retractor penis m.

Venous plexus dorsal to penis

Bulbospongiosus m.

Penile urethra

Corpus cavernosum
penis

Rectus abdominis m.

Convoluted portion of
ductus deferens

Internal prepuce

Glans penis

Tail of epididymis

Urethral sinus

Urethral process

Body of epididymis

External urethral orifice

Fossa glandis

Scrotum

Internal prepuce

External prepuce
(sheath)

Head of epididymis

Left testis

**22**

**PLATE 1.21**    Relations of the reproductive organs of the stallion.
Median section, right lateral view. m = muscle

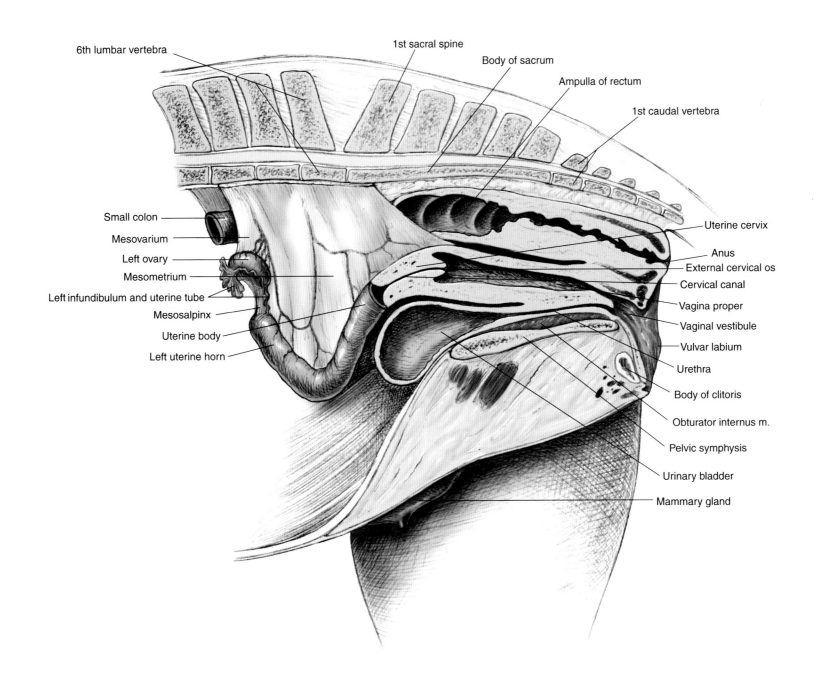

6th lumbar vertebra

1st sacral spine

Body of sacrum

Ampulla of rectum

1st caudal vertebra

Small colon

Mesovarium

Left ovary

Mesometrium

Left infundibulum and uterine tube

Mesosalpinx

Uterine body

Left uterine horn

Uterine cervix

Anus

External cervical os

Cervical canal

Vagina proper

Vaginal vestibule

Vulvar labium

Urethra

Body of clitoris

Obturator internus m.

Pelvic symphysis

Urinary bladder

Mammary gland

**PLATE 1.22** Relations of the reproductive organs of the mare. Partial median section.
Left lateral view. m = muscle

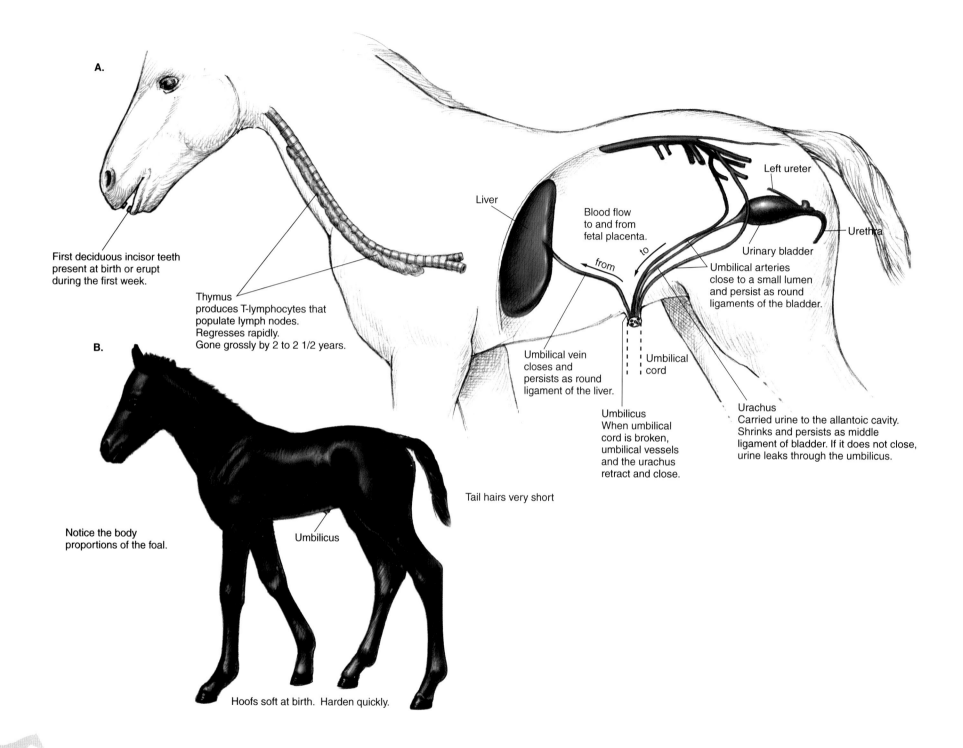

**A.**

First deciduous incisor teeth present at birth or erupt during the first week.

Thymus produces T-lymphocytes that populate lymph nodes. Regresses rapidly. Gone grossly by 2 to 2 1/2 years.

Liver

Blood flow to and from fetal placenta.

*from*

*to*

Left ureter

Urethra

Urinary bladder

Umbilical arteries close to a small lumen and persist as round ligaments of the bladder.

Umbilical vein closes and persists as round ligament of the liver.

Umbilical cord

Umbilicus
When umbilical cord is broken, umbilical vessels and the urachus retract and close.

Urachus
Carried urine to the allantoic cavity. Shrinks and persists as middle ligament of bladder. If it does not close, urine leaks through the umbilicus.

Tail hairs very short

**B.**

Notice the body proportions of the foal.

Umbilicus

Hoofs soft at birth. Harden quickly.

24

**PLATE 1.23** Neonatal organs of the foal. Left lateral view.

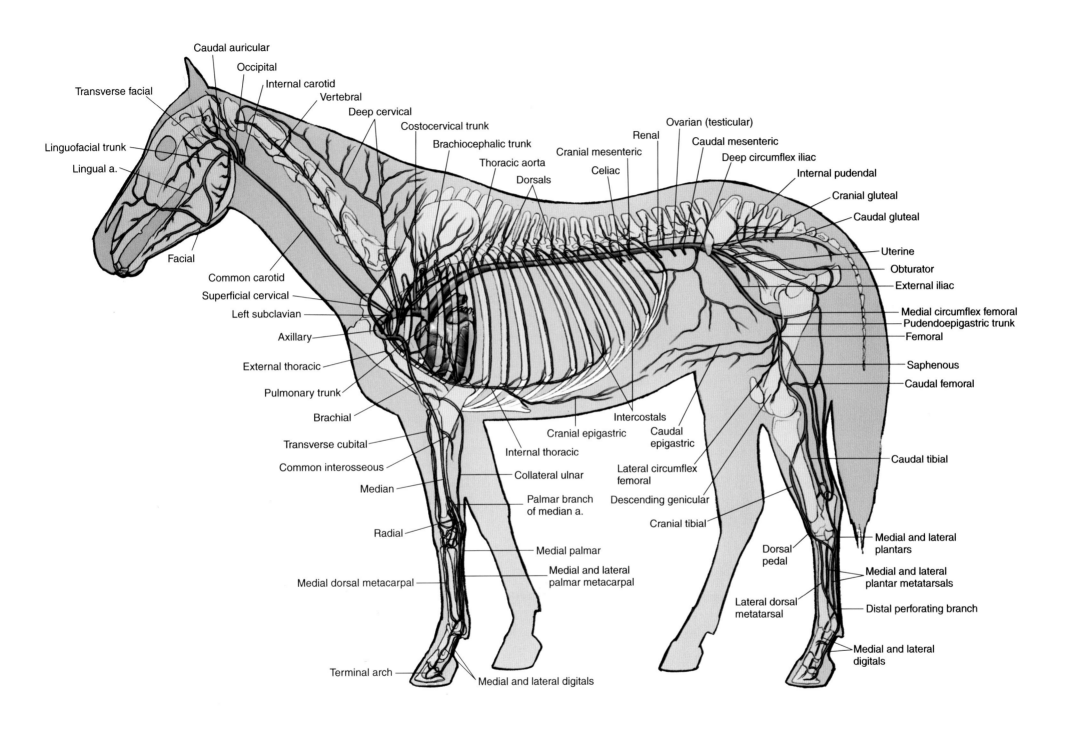

Caudal auricular
Occipital
Internal carotid
Vertebral
Deep cervical
Costocervical trunk
Brachiocephalic trunk
Thoracic aorta
Dorsals
Cranial mesenteric
Celiac
Renal
Ovarian (testicular)
Caudal mesenteric
Deep circumflex iliac
Internal pudendal
Cranial gluteal
Caudal gluteal
Transverse facial
Linguofacial trunk
Lingual a.
Facial
Common carotid
Superficial cervical
Left subclavian
Axillary
External thoracic
Pulmonary trunk
Brachial
Transverse cubital
Common interosseous
Median
Radial
Medial dorsal metacarpal
Terminal arch
Medial and lateral digitals
Internal thoracic
Cranial epigastric
Collateral ulnar
Palmar branch
of median a.
Medial palmar
Medial and lateral
palmar metacarpal
Intercostals
Caudal
epigastric
Lateral circumflex
femoral
Descending genicular
Cranial tibial
Dorsal
pedal
Lateral dorsal
metatarsal
Uterine
Obturator
External iliac
Medial circumflex femoral
Pudendoepigastric trunk
Femoral
Saphenous
Caudal femoral
Caudal tibial
Medial and lateral
plantars
Medial and lateral
plantar metatarsals
Distal perforating branch
Medial and lateral
digitals

25

**PLATE 1.24**   Major arteries of the mare.  Left lateral view. a = artery

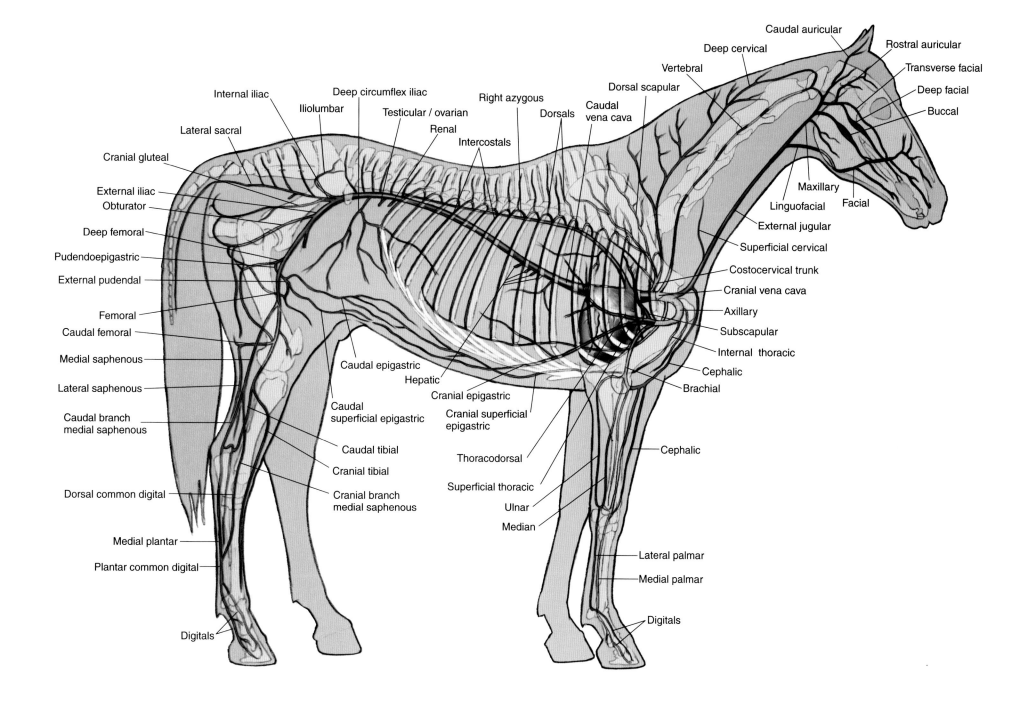

**PLATE 1.25**   Major veins of the stallion. Portal system excluded.   Right lateral view.

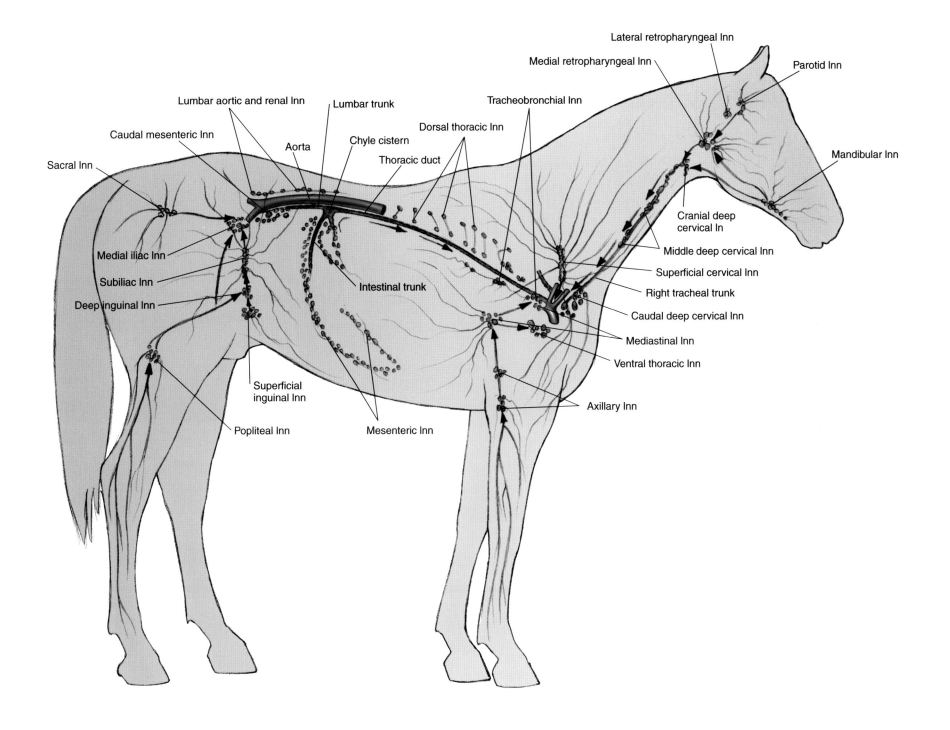

**PLATE 1.26** Lymph nodes and vessels of the horse. Right lateral view. *Arrows* indicate the flow of lymph. Lymph node groups in the horse consist of up to dozens of lymph nodes ranging in size from a few millimeters to 2 centimeters in diameter. ln = lymph node

27

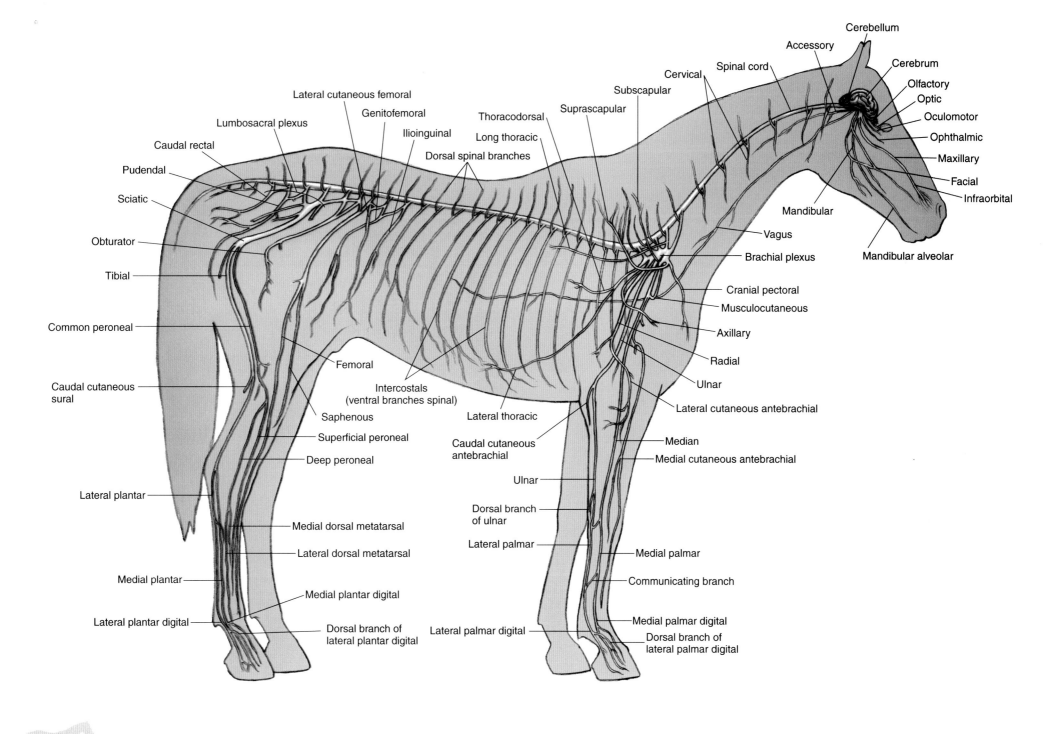

**PLATE 1.27** Central and somatic nervous system of the stallion. Right lateral view.

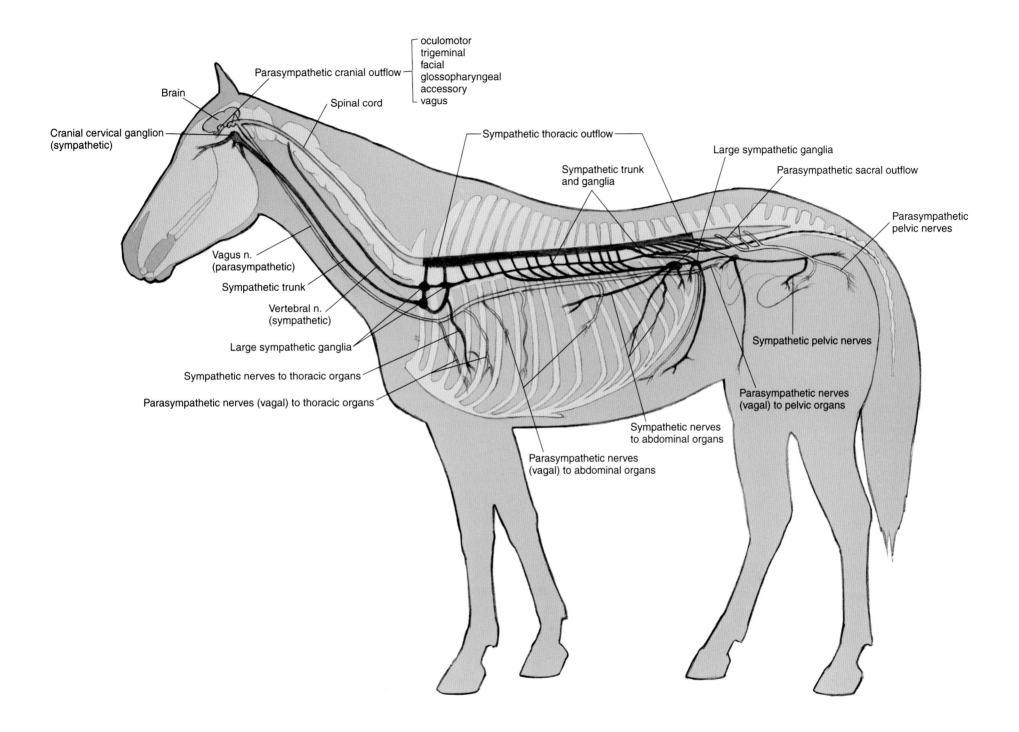

oculomotor
trigeminal
facial
glossopharyngeal
accessory
vagus

Parasympathetic cranial outflow

Brain

Spinal cord

Cranial cervical ganglion
(sympathetic)

Sympathetic thoracic outflow

Large sympathetic ganglia

Sympathetic trunk
and ganglia

Parasympathetic sacral outflow

Parasympathetic
pelvic nerves

Vagus n.
(parasympathetic)

Sympathetic trunk

Vertebral n.
(sympathetic)

Large sympathetic ganglia

Sympathetic nerves to thoracic organs

Parasympathetic nerves (vagal) to thoracic organs

Sympathetic pelvic nerves

Parasympathetic nerves
(vagal) to pelvic organs

Sympathetic nerves
to abdominal organs

Parasympathetic nerves
(vagal) to abdominal organs

29

**PLATE 1.28**  Autonomic nervous system of the mare.  Left lateral view. n = nerve

# SECTION 2 THE OX (*Bos taurus,* also *Bos indicus*)

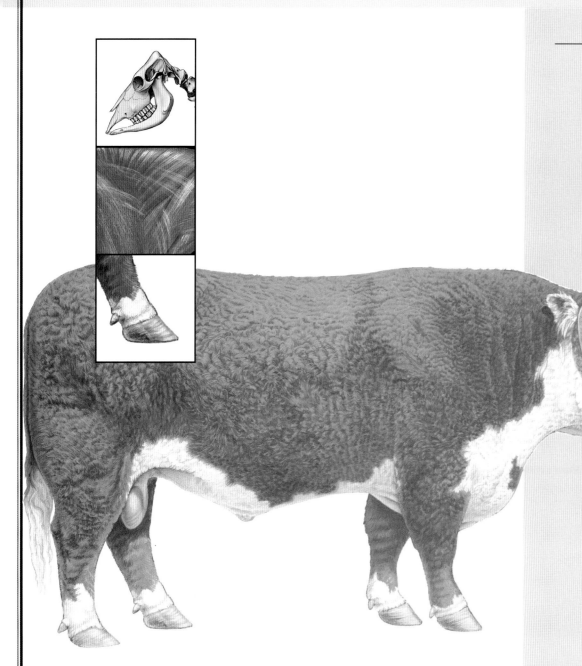

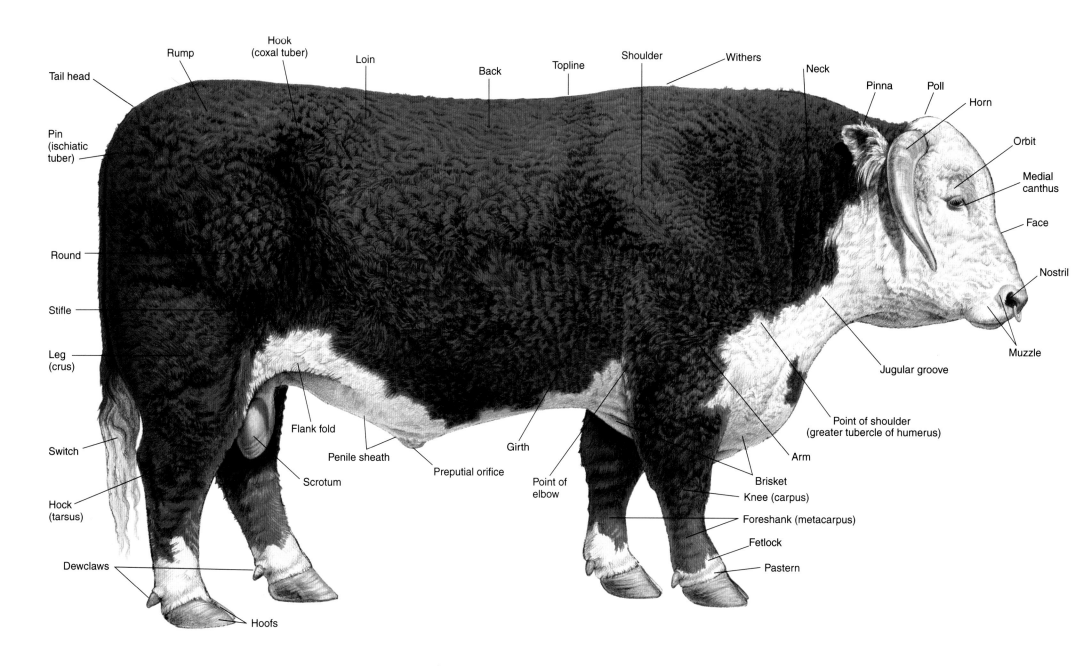

**PLATE 2.1** Right lateral view of a beef bull.

32

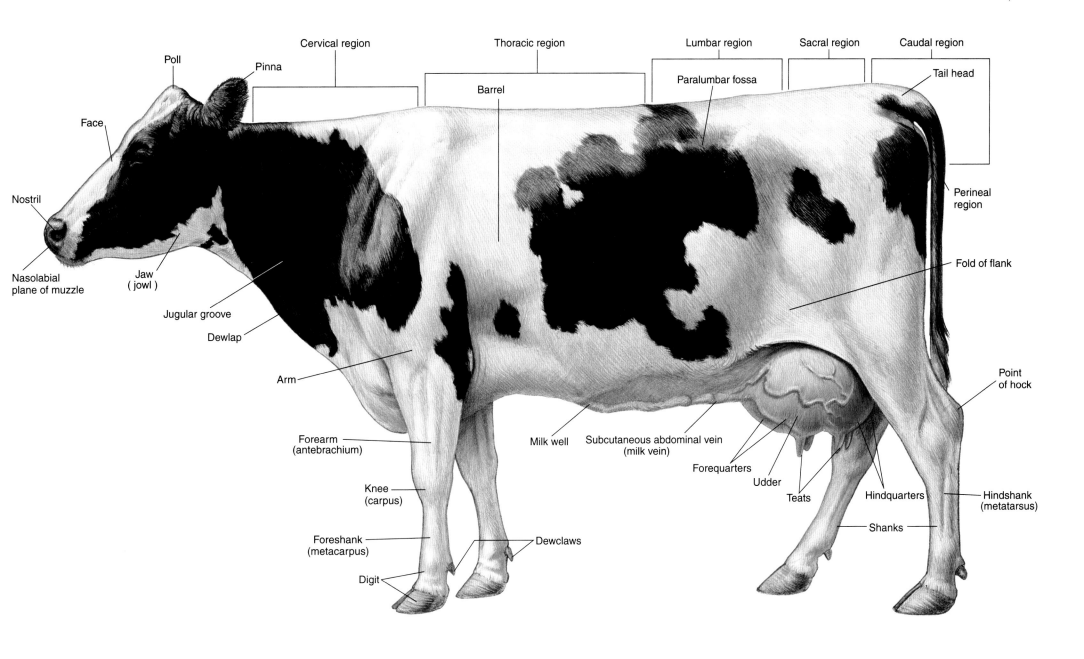

Cervical region Thoracic region Lumbar region Sacral region Caudal region

Poll
Pinna
Face
Barrel
Paralumbar fossa
Tail head
Nostril
Nasolabial
plane of muzzle
Jaw
( jowl )
Jugular groove
Dewlap
Arm
Perineal
region
Fold of flank
Forearm
(antebrachium)
Milk well
Subcutaneous abdominal vein
(milk vein)
Point
of hock
Knee
(carpus)
Forequarters
Udder
Hindquarters
Hindshank
(metatarsus)
Foreshank
(metacarpus)
Dewclaws
Teats
Shanks
Digit

**33**

**PLATE 2.2**   Left lateral view of a dairy cow. Dorsal vertebral regions indicated.

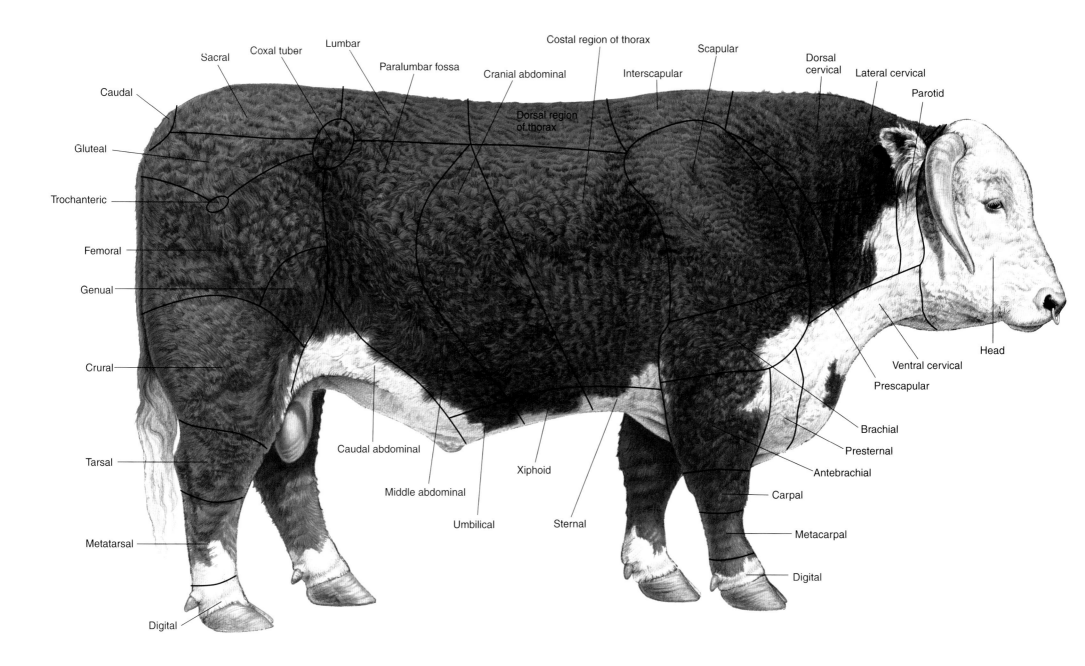

Caudal

Sacral

Coxal tuber

Lumbar

Paralumbar fossa

Cranial abdominal

Costal region of thorax

Dorsal region of thorax

Interscapular

Scapular

Dorsal cervical

Lateral cervical

Parotid

Gluteal

Trochanteric

Femoral

Genual

Crural

Tarsal

Metatarsal

Digital

Caudal abdominal

Middle abdominal

Umbilical

Xiphoid

Sternal

Head

Ventral cervical

Prescapular

Brachial

Presternal

Antebrachial

Carpal

Metacarpal

Digital

**34**

**PLATE 2.3**   Body regions of the ox. Right lateral view.

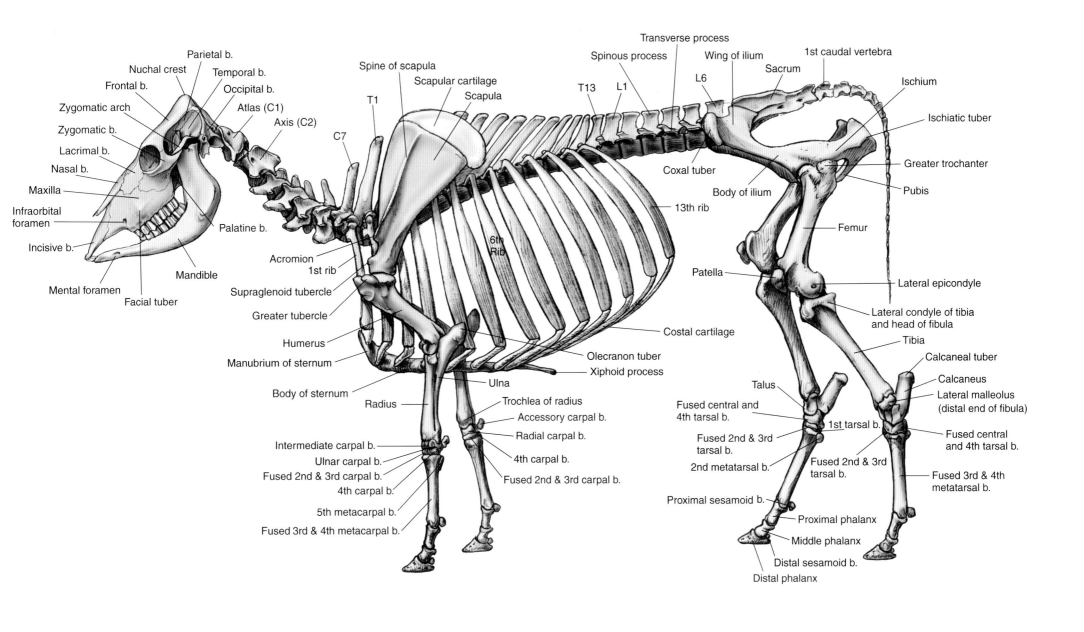

Nuchal crest
Parietal b.
Frontal b.
Temporal b.
Zygomatic arch
Occipital b.
Zygomatic b.
Atlas (C1)
Lacrimal b.
Axis (C2)
Nasal b.
Maxilla
Infraorbital foramen
Palatine b.
Incisive b.
Mandible
Mental foramen
Facial tuber

Spine of scapula
Scapular cartilage
Scapula
T1
C7
Acromion
1st rib
Supraglenoid tubercle
Greater tubercle
Humerus
Manubrium of sternum
Body of sternum
Radius
Trochlea of radius
Accessory carpal b.
Radial carpal b.
4th carpal b.
Fused 2nd & 3rd carpal b.
Intermediate carpal b.
Ulnar carpal b.
Fused 2nd & 3rd carpal b.
4th carpal b.
5th metacarpal b.
Fused 3rd & 4th metacarpal b.

Transverse process
Spinous process
Wing of ilium
1st caudal vertebra
Sacrum
T13
L1
L6
Ischium
Ischiatic tuber
Coxal tuber
Body of ilium
Greater trochanter
Pubis
13th rib
Femur
6th Rib
Patella
Lateral epicondyle
Lateral condyle of tibia and head of fibula
Costal cartilage
Tibia
Olecranon tuber
Xiphoid process
Calcaneal tuber
Ulna
Talus
Calcaneus
Fused central and 4th tarsal b.
Lateral malleolus (distal end of fibula)
1st tarsal b.
Fused 2nd & 3rd tarsal b.
Fused central and 4th tarsal b.
2nd metatarsal b.
Fused 2nd & 3rd tarsal b.
Fused 3rd & 4th metatarsal b.
Proximal sesamoid b.
Proximal phalanx
Middle phalanx
Distal sesamoid b.
Distal phalanx

35

**PLATE 2.4**   Skeleton of the ox. Left lateral view. C = cervical vertebra, T = thoracic vertebra, L = lumbar vertebra, b = bone

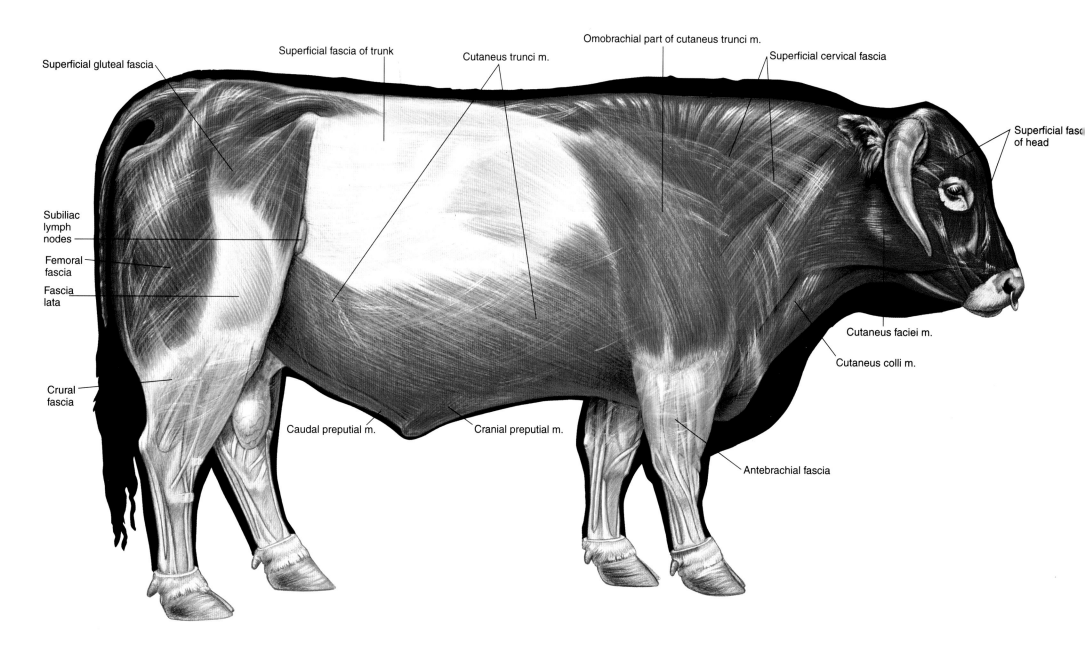

Superficial gluteal fascia

Superficial fascia of trunk

Cutaneus trunci m.

Omobrachial part of cutaneus trunci m.

Superficial cervical fascia

Superficial fascia of head

Subiliac lymph nodes

Femoral fascia

Fascia lata

Crural fascia

Caudal preputial m.

Cranial preputial m.

Cutaneus faciei m.

Cutaneus colli m.

Antebrachial fascia

**PLATE 2.5**   Cutaneous muscles and major fasciae of the bull. Right lateral view. n = nerve, m = muscle

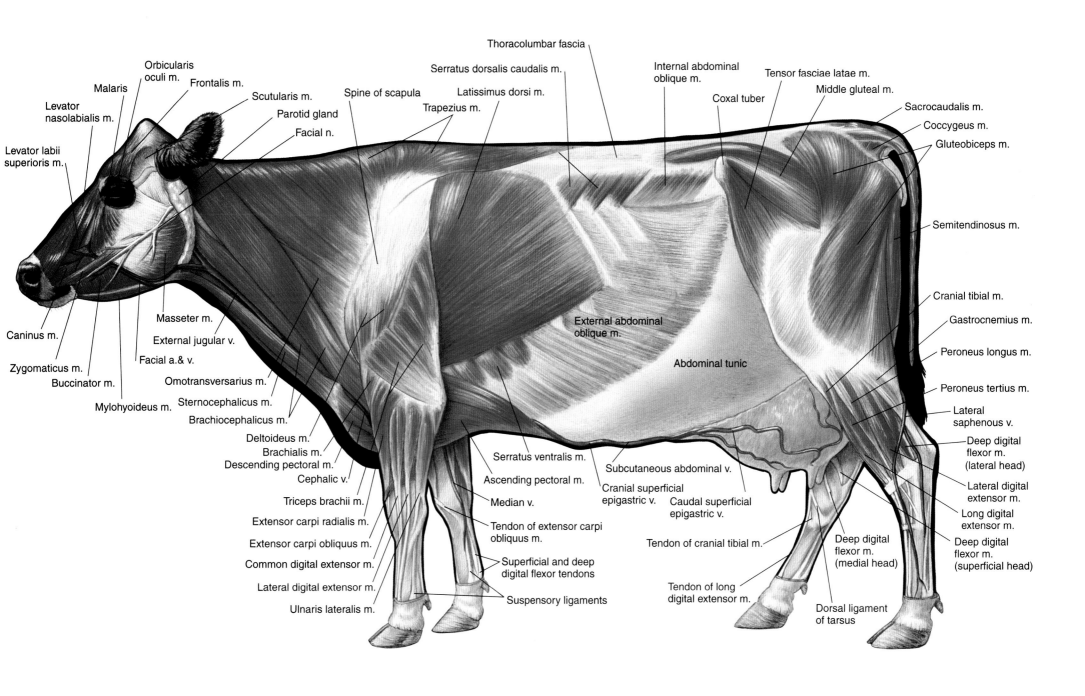

**PLATE 2.6** Superficial muscles and veins of the cow. Left lateral view.
m = muscle, v = vein, a = artery, n = nerve

37

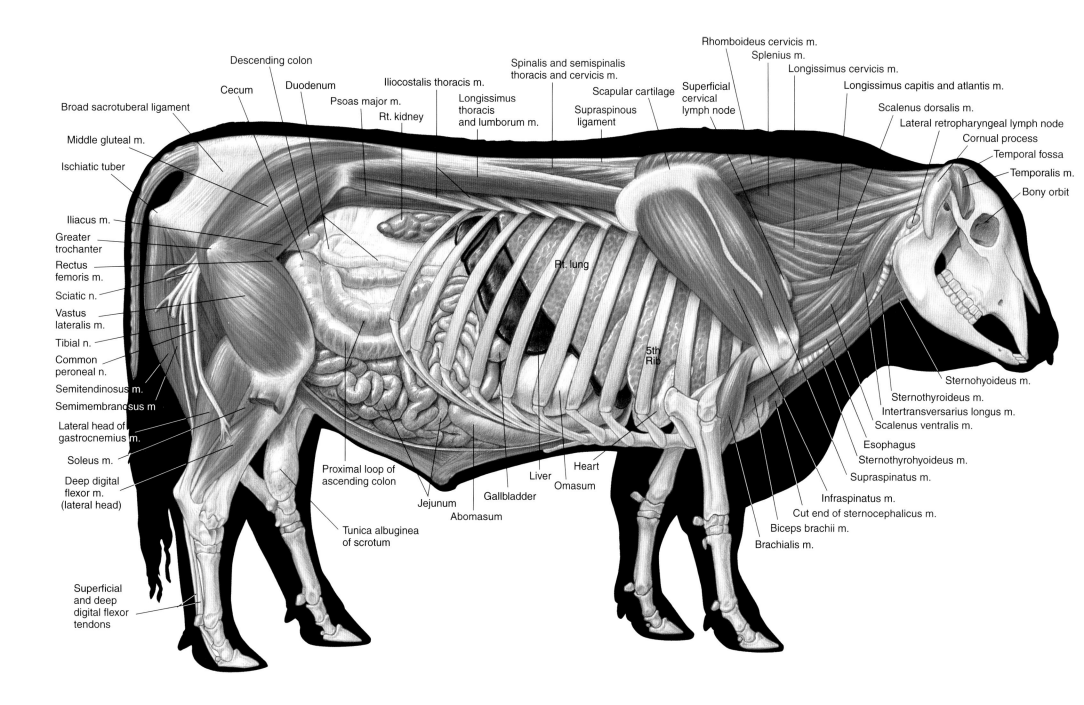

Descending colon

Cecum

Duodenum

Broad sacrotuberal ligament

Psoas major m.

Rt. kidney

Iliocostalis thoracis m.

Longissimus thoracis and lumborum m.

Spinalis and semispinalis thoracis and cervicis m.

Scapular cartilage

Supraspinous ligament

Superficial cervical lymph node

Rhomboideus cervicis m.

Splenius m.

Longissimus cervicis m.

Longissimus capitis and atlantis m.

Scalenus dorsalis m.

Lateral retropharyngeal lymph node

Cornual process

Temporal fossa

Temporalis m.

Bony orbit

Middle gluteal m.

Ischiatic tuber

Iliacus m.

Greater trochanter

Rectus femoris m.

Sciatic n.

Vastus lateralis m.

Tibial n.

Common peroneal n.

Semitendinosus m.

Semimembranosus m

Lateral head of gastrocnemius m.

Soleus m.

Deep digital flexor m. (lateral head)

Superficial and deep digital flexor tendons

Rt. lung

5th Rib

Proximal loop of ascending colon

Jejunum

Tunica albuginea of scrotum

Abomasum

Gallbladder

Liver

Omasum

Heart

Sternohyoideus m.

Sternothyroideus m.

Intertransversarius longus m.

Scalenus ventralis m.

Esophagus

Sternothyrohyoideus m.

Supraspinatus m.

Infraspinatus m.

Cut end of sternocephalicus m.

Biceps brachii m.

Brachialis m.

38

**PLATE 2.7**   Deep cervical muscles and *in situ* viscera of the bull. Greater omentum removed. Right lateral view. m = muscle, n = nerve

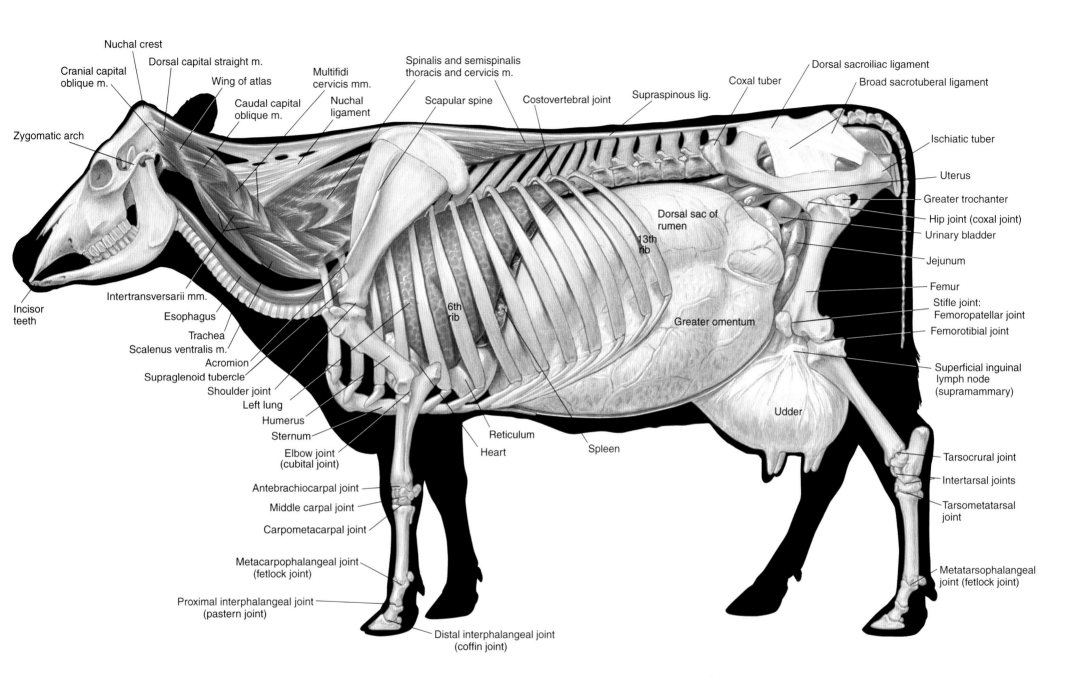

**PLATE 2.8** Deep cervical muscles, major joints, *in situ* viscera, and udder of the cow.
Left lateral view. m = muscle, lig = ligament

39

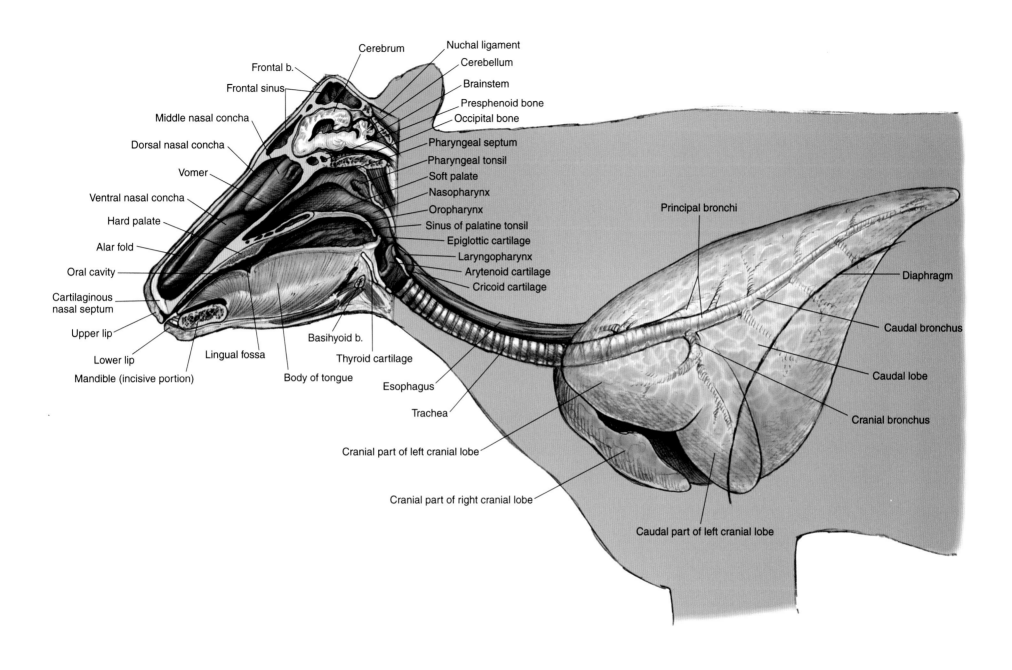

Cerebrum
Frontal b.
Frontal sinus
Middle nasal concha
Dorsal nasal concha
Vomer
Ventral nasal concha
Hard palate
Alar fold
Oral cavity
Cartilaginous nasal septum
Upper lip
Lower lip
Mandible (incisive portion)
Lingual fossa
Body of tongue
Basihyoid b.
Thyroid cartilage
Esophagus
Trachea
Cranial part of left cranial lobe
Cranial part of right cranial lobe
Caudal part of left cranial lobe

Nuchal ligament
Cerebellum
Brainstem
Presphenoid bone
Occipital bone
Pharyngeal septum
Pharyngeal tonsil
Soft palate
Nasopharynx
Oropharynx
Sinus of palatine tonsil
Epiglottic cartilage
Laryngopharynx
Arytenoid cartilage
Cricoid cartilage

Principal bronchi
Diaphragm
Caudal bronchus
Caudal lobe
Cranial bronchus

**40**

**PLATE 2.9**  Median section of the head and left lateral view of the
respiratory system of the ox. b = bone

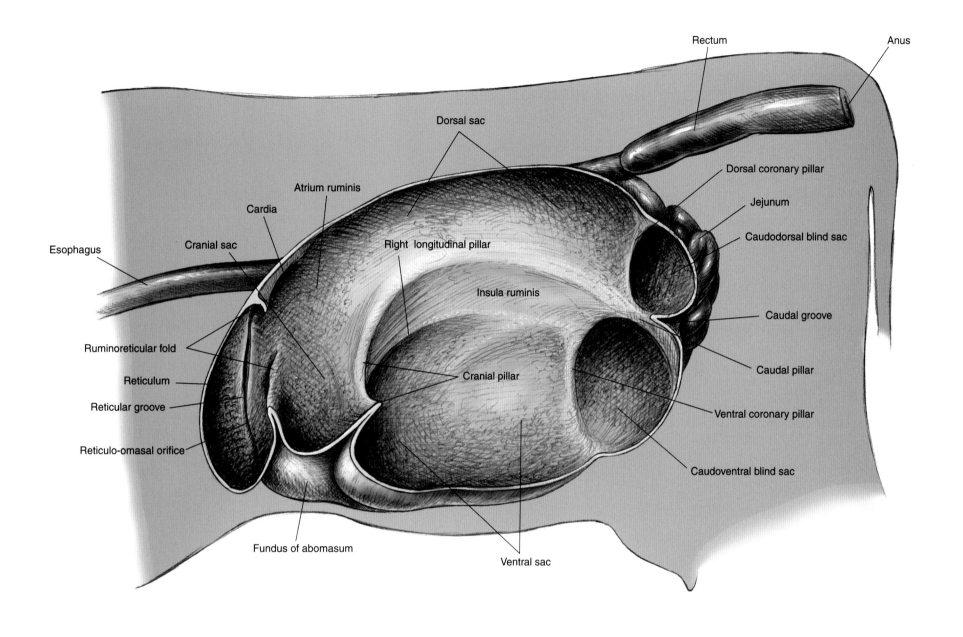

Rectum

Anus

Dorsal sac

Dorsal coronary pillar

Atrium ruminis

Jejunum

Cardia

Caudodorsal blind sac

Esophagus

Cranial sac

Right  longitudinal pillar

Insula ruminis

Caudal groove

Ruminoreticular fold

Reticulum

Cranial pillar

Caudal pillar

Reticular groove

Ventral coronary pillar

Reticulo-omasal orifice

Caudoventral blind sac

Fundus of abomasum

Ventral sac

**PLATE 2.10** Interior of the rumen and reticulum of the cow. Left lateral view.

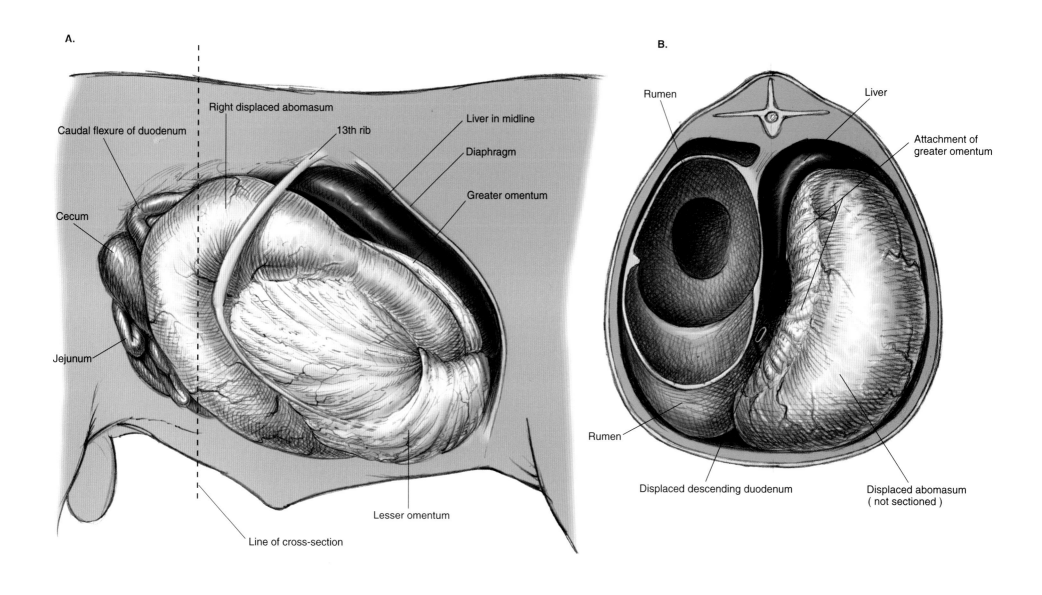

**A.**

Caudal flexure of duodenum

Right displaced abomasum

13th rib

Liver in midline

Diaphragm

Greater omentum

Cecum

Jejunum

Lesser omentum

Line of cross-section

**B.**

Rumen

Liver

Attachment of greater omentum

Rumen

Displaced descending duodenum

Displaced abomasum ( not sectioned )

**PLATE 2.11**  Clinical condition: Right volvulus of the abomasum in a bull. **A.** Right lateral view.
**B.** Cross-section. Caudocranial view.  This problem occurs in cattle of varying types and
ages.  The long axis of the abomasum rotates dorsad and caudad, moving the
greater curvature of the abomasum counterclockwise and toward the
pelvis.  This abnormal configuration displaces the liver mediad
and draws the pyloric antrum and duodenum around
the cranial aspect of the omasum.

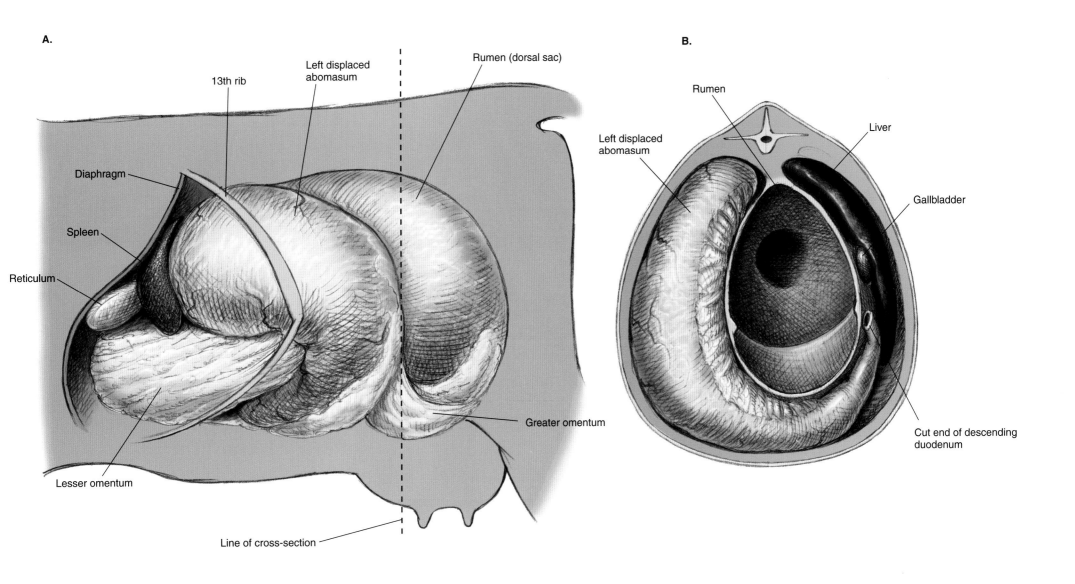

**A.**

13th rib

Left displaced abomasum

Rumen (dorsal sac)

Diaphragm

Spleen

Reticulum

Lesser omentum

Line of cross-section

Greater omentum

**B.**

Rumen

Left displaced abomasum

Liver

Gallbladder

Cut end of descending duodenum

**PLATE 2.12**  Clinical condition: Left displacement of the abomasum in a cow. **A.** Left lateral view.
**B.** Cross-section. Caudocranial view. This problem can occur commonly in lactating dairy
cattle during the first month postpartum and less frequently during other times
or in other types of cattle.  The gas-filled abomasum moves to the left and
dorsad in the abdomen.  It displaces the partially filled rumen
mediad and distorts the normal position and orientation of
the reticulum, omasum, and cranial rumen.

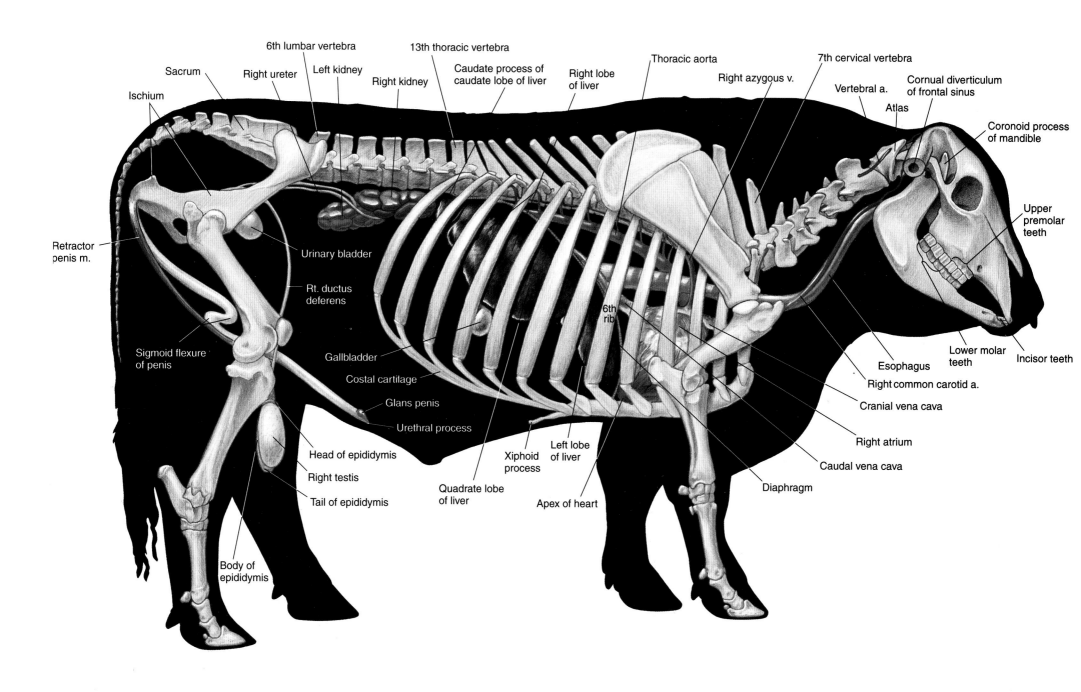

6th lumbar vertebra

13th thoracic vertebra

Sacrum

Right ureter    Left kidney

Thoracic aorta

7th cervical vertebra

Ischium

Right kidney

Caudate process of
caudate lobe of liver

Right lobe
of liver

Right azygous v.

Vertebral a.

Cornual diverticulum
of frontal sinus

Atlas

Coronoid process
of mandible

Retractor
penis m.

Urinary bladder

Upper
premolar
teeth

Rt. ductus
deferens

Sigmoid flexure
of penis

6th
rib

Gallbladder

Esophagus

Costal cartilage

Lower molar
teeth

Incisor teeth

Glans penis

Right common carotid a.

Urethral process

Cranial vena cava

Head of epididymis

Left lobe
of liver

Right atrium

Right testis

Xiphoid
process

Caudal vena cava

Tail of epididymis

Quadrate lobe
of liver

Apex of heart

Diaphragm

Body of
epididymis

44

**PLATE 2.13**   Reproductive organs, urinary organs, liver, heart, and adjacent major
vessels related to the skeleton of the bull. Stomach, intestines, and lungs are
removed. Right lateral view. a = artery, v = vein, m = muscle

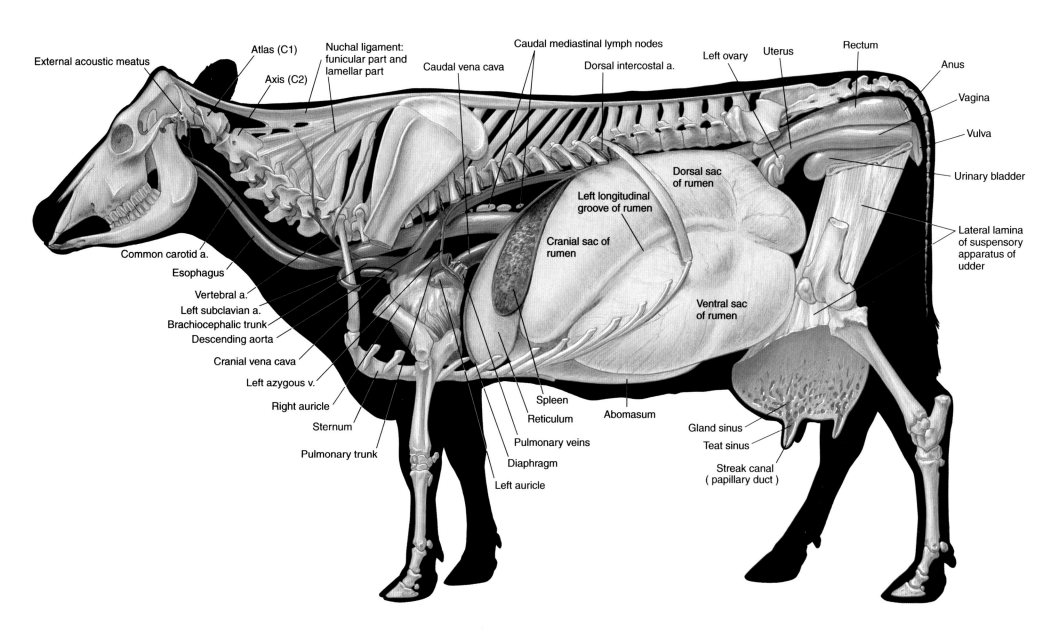

External acoustic meatus

Atlas (C1)

Axis (C2)

Nuchal ligament:
funicular part and
lamellar part

Caudal vena cava

Caudal mediastinal lymph nodes

Dorsal intercostal a.

Left ovary

Uterus

Rectum

Anus

Vagina

Vulva

Urinary bladder

Lateral lamina
of suspensory
apparatus of
udder

Common carotid a.

Esophagus

Vertebral a.

Left subclavian a.

Brachiocephalic trunk

Descending aorta

Cranial vena cava

Left azygous v.

Right auricle

Sternum

Pulmonary trunk

Dorsal sac
of rumen

Left longitudinal
groove of rumen

Cranial sac of
rumen

Ventral sac
of rumen

Spleen

Reticulum

Abomasum

Pulmonary veins

Diaphragm

Left auricle

Gland sinus

Teat sinus

Streak canal
( papillary duct )

**PLATE 2.14**   Heart and adjacent major vessels, abdominal and pelvic viscera,
and udder (mammary glands) of the cow. Lungs and intestines are
removed. Left lateral view. v = vein, a = artery

45

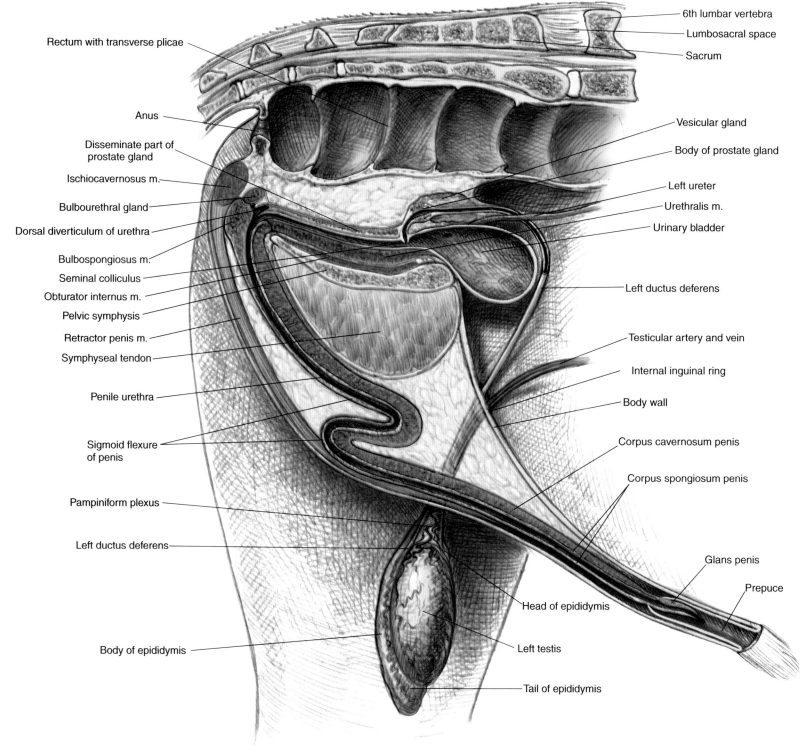

46

**PLATE 2.15** Relations of the reproductive organs of the bull. Median section. m = muscle

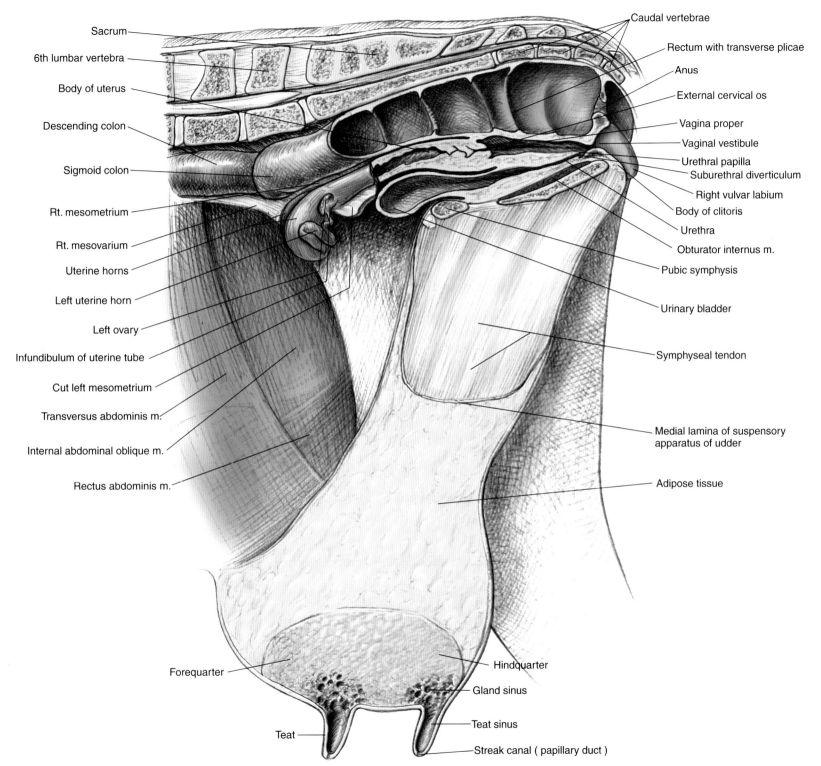

Sacrum

6th lumbar vertebra

Body of uterus

Descending colon

Sigmoid colon

Rt. mesometrium

Rt. mesovarium

Uterine horns

Left uterine horn

Left ovary

Infundibulum of uterine tube

Cut left mesometrium

Transversus abdominis m.

Internal abdominal oblique m.

Rectus abdominis m.

Forequarter

Teat

Caudal vertebrae

Rectum with transverse plicae

Anus

External cervical os

Vagina proper

Vaginal vestibule

Urethral papilla

Suburethral diverticulum

Right vulvar labium

Body of clitoris

Urethra

Obturator internus m.

Pubic symphysis

Urinary bladder

Symphyseal tendon

Medial lamina of suspensory apparatus of udder

Adipose tissue

Hindquarter

Gland sinus

Teat sinus

Streak canal ( papillary duct )

47

**PLATE 2.16**   Relations of the reproductive organs of the cow. Median section. m = muscle

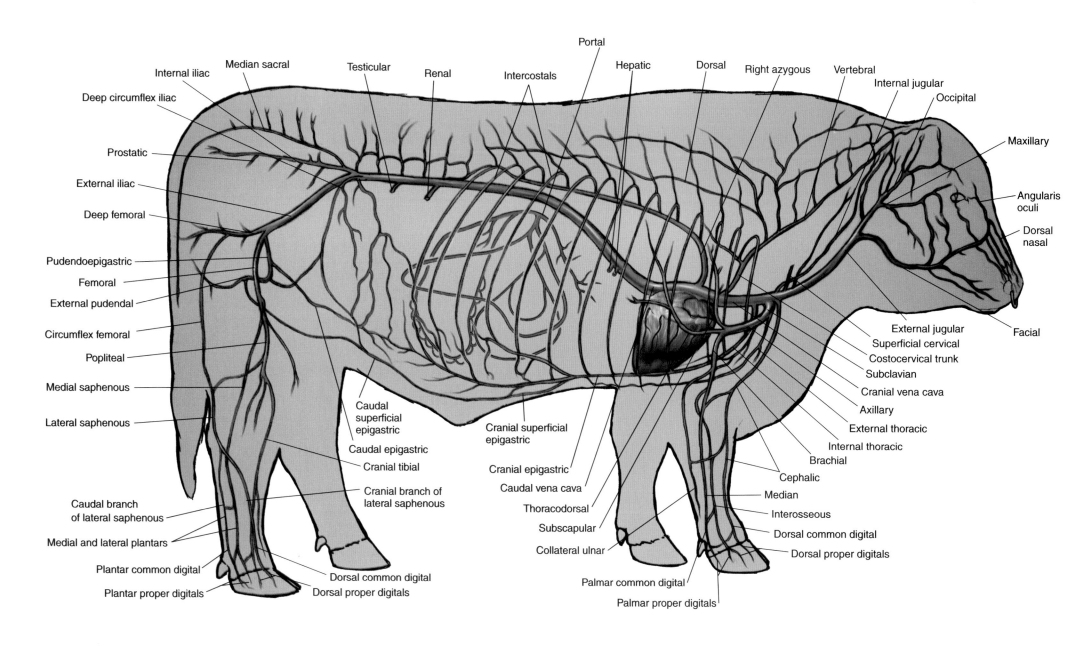

**PLATE 2.17**  Major veins of the bull. Right lateral view.

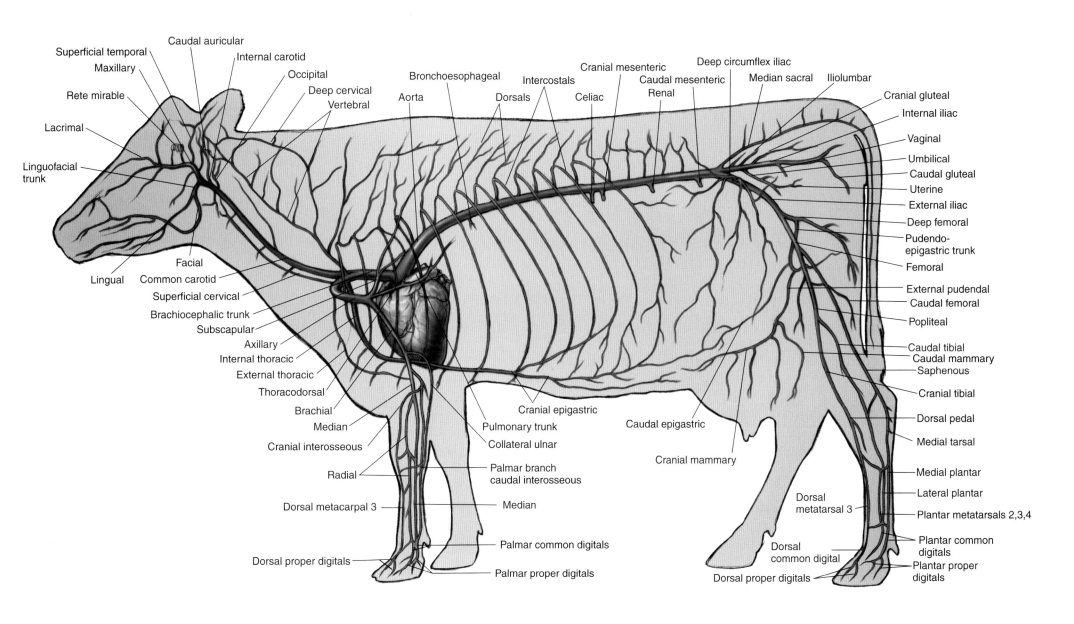

**PLATE 2.18** Major arteries of the cow. Left lateral view.

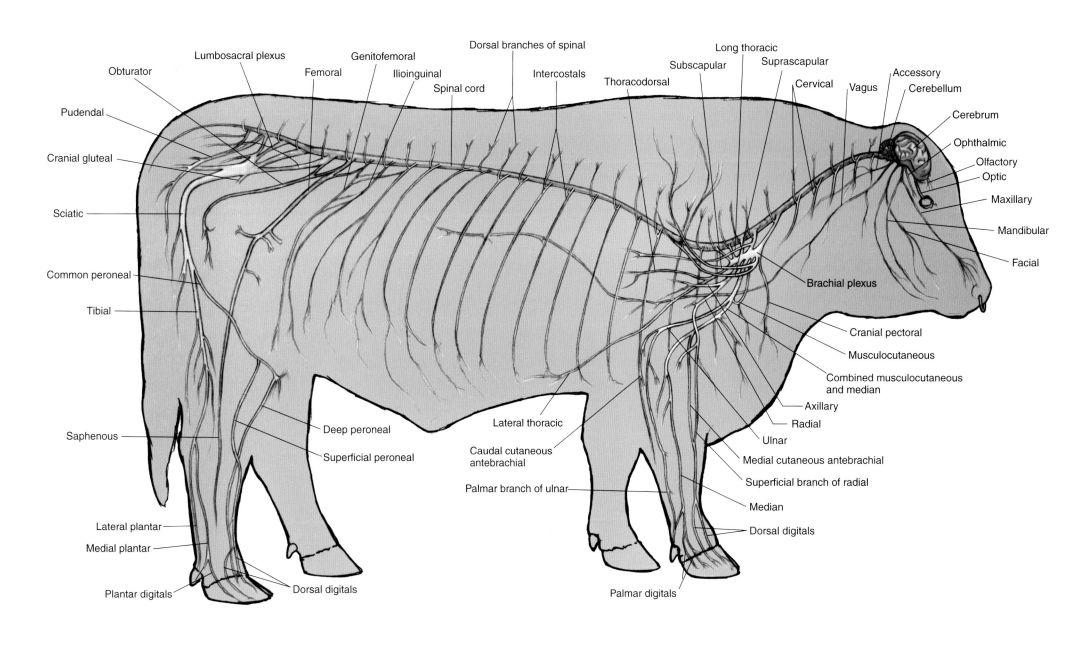

**PLATE 2.19** Central nervous system and principal nerves of the peripheral nervous system of the bull. Right lateral view.

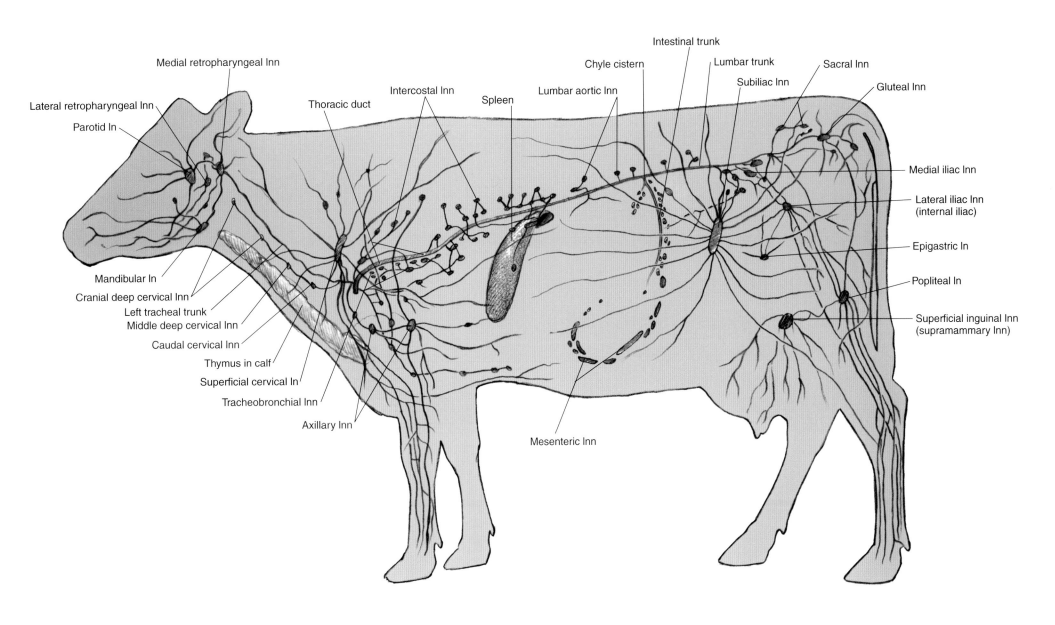

**PLATE 2.20** Significant lymphatic organs of the cow. Left lateral view. ln = lymph node

Medial retropharyngeal lnn

Lateral retropharyngeal lnn

Parotid ln

Intestinal trunk

Chyle cistern

Lumbar trunk

Sacral lnn

Intercostal lnn

Thoracic duct

Spleen

Lumbar aortic lnn

Subiliac lnn

Gluteal lnn

Medial iliac lnn

Lateral iliac lnn
(internal iliac)

Epigastric ln

Popliteal ln

Superficial inguinal lnn
(supramammary lnn)

Mandibular ln

Cranial deep cervical lnn

Left tracheal trunk

Middle deep cervical lnn

Caudal cervical lnn

Thymus in calf

Superficial cervical ln

Tracheobronchial lnn

Axillary lnn

Mesenteric lnn

51

# SECTION 3 THE SHEEP *(Ovis aries)*

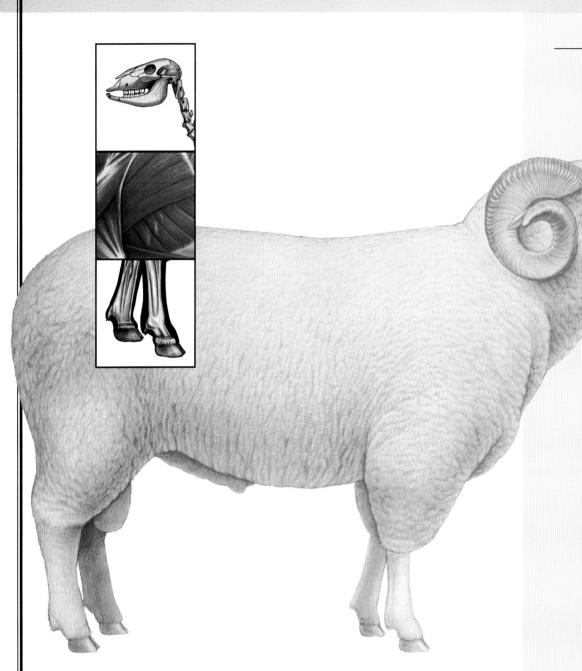

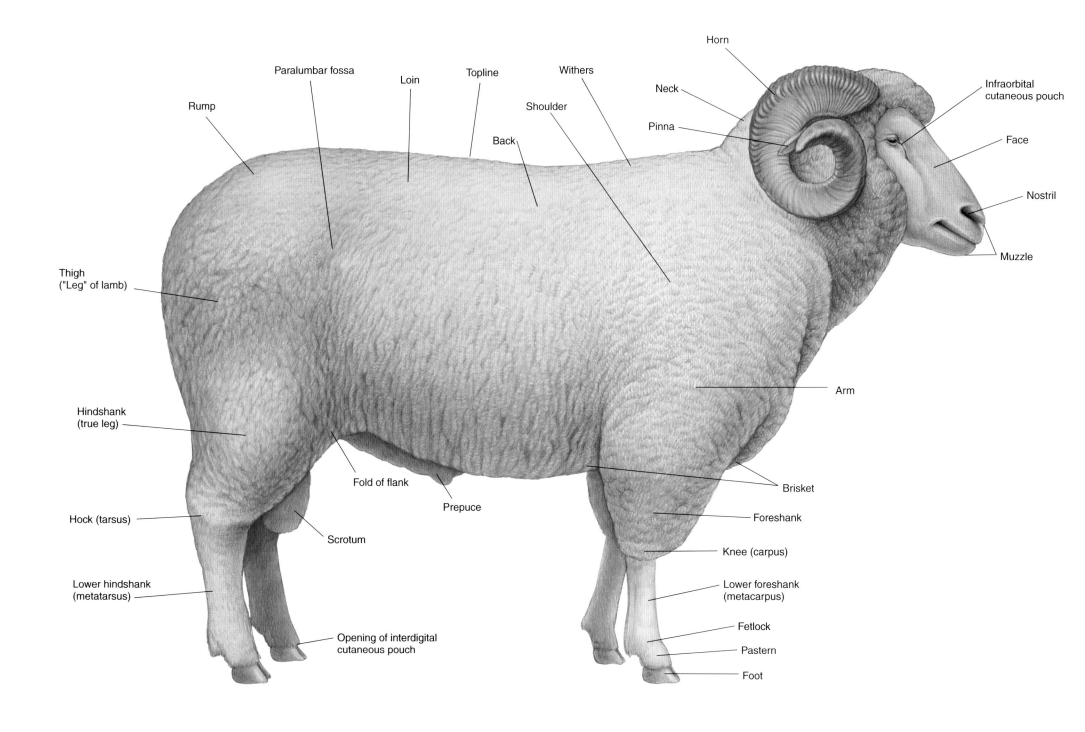

Rump

Paralumbar fossa

Loin

Topline

Withers

Horn

Neck

Infraorbital
cutaneous pouch

Shoulder

Pinna

Face

Back

Nostril

Thigh
("Leg" of lamb)

Muzzle

Arm

Hindshank
(true leg)

Fold of flank

Brisket

Prepuce

Foreshank

Hock (tarsus)

Scrotum

Knee (carpus)

Lower hindshank
(metatarsus)

Lower foreshank
(metacarpus)

Fetlock

Pastern

Opening of interdigital
cutaneous pouch

Foot

**54**

**PLATE 3.1**   Right lateral view of a ram.

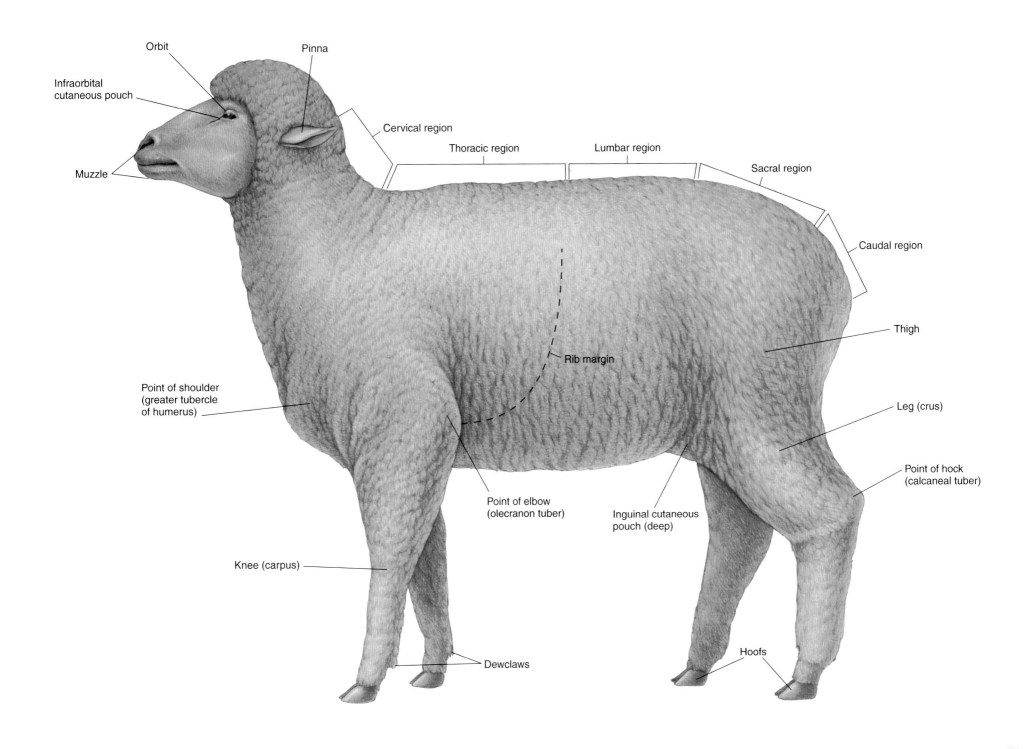

Orbit

Pinna

Infraorbital
cutaneous pouch

Cervical region

Thoracic region

Lumbar region

Sacral region

Muzzle

Caudal region

Rib margin

Thigh

Point of shoulder
(greater tubercle
of humerus)

Leg (crus)

Point of hock
(calcaneal tuber)

Point of elbow
(olecranon tuber)

Inguinal cutaneous
pouch (deep)

Knee (carpus)

Hoofs

Dewclaws

**55**

**PLATE 3.2**  Left lateral view of an ewe.

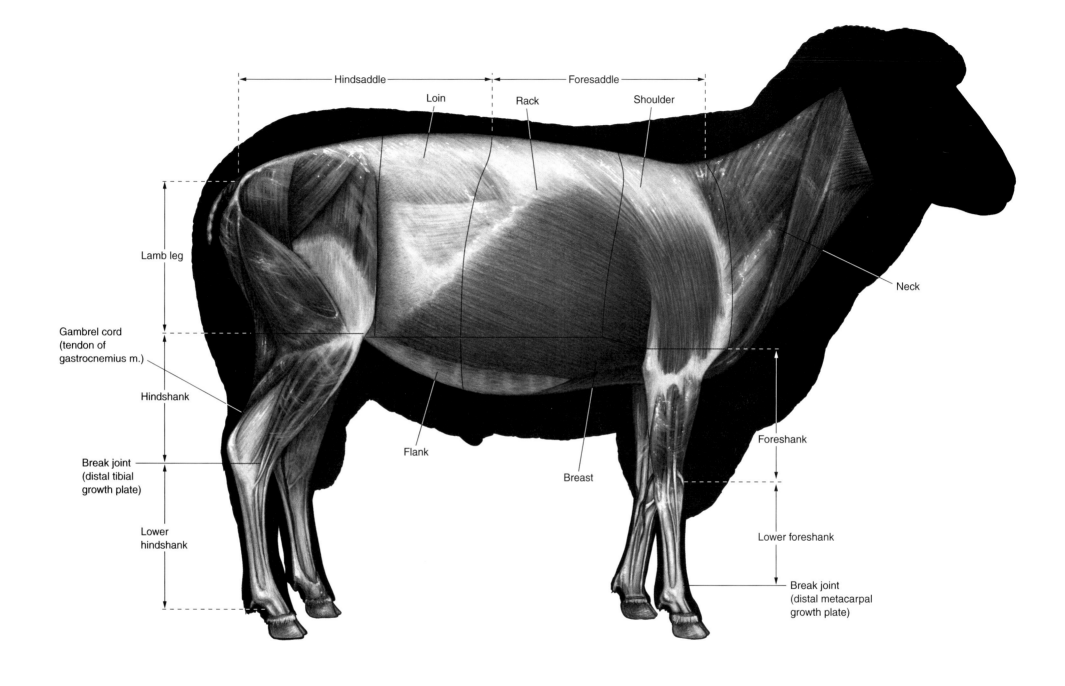

Hindsaddle · Foresaddle

Loin · Rack · Shoulder

Lamb leg

Gambrel cord
(tendon of
gastrocnemius m.)

Hindshank

Break joint
(distal tibial
growth plate)

Lower
hindshank

Flank

Breast

Neck

Foreshank

Lower foreshank

Break joint
(distal metacarpal
growth plate)

**PLATE 3.3**   Carcass cuts of the lamb. m = muscle

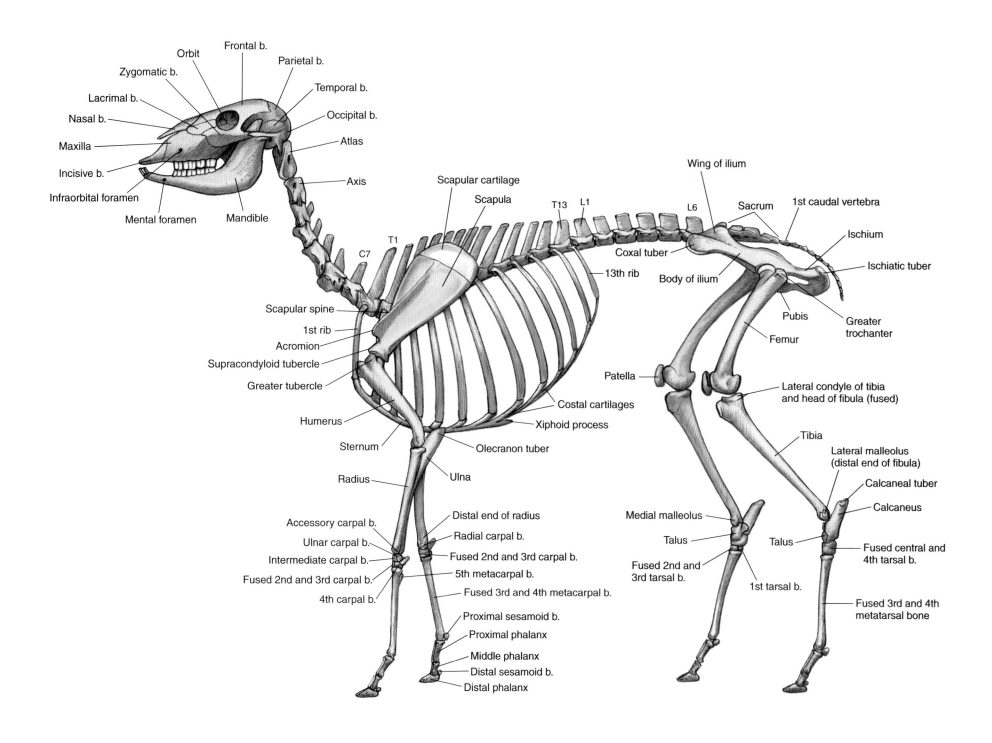

**PLATE 3.4** Skeleton of the sheep. b = bone, C = cervical vertebra,
T = thoracic vertebra, L = lumbar vertebra

57

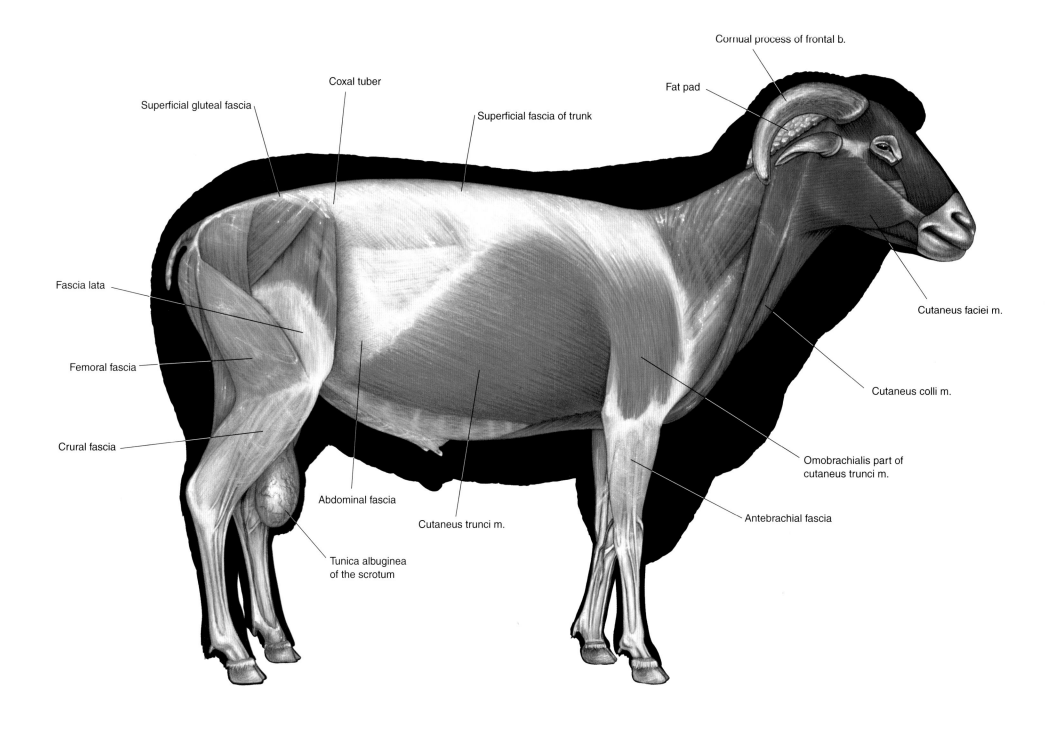

Cornual process of frontal b.

Coxal tuber

Superficial fascia of trunk

Fat pad

Superficial gluteal fascia

Fascia lata

Femoral fascia

Crural fascia

Cutaneus faciei m.

Cutaneus colli m.

Omobrachialis part of
cutaneus trunci m.

Abdominal fascia

Cutaneus trunci m.

Antebrachial fascia

Tunica albuginea
of the scrotum

**58**

**PLATE 3.5**   Cutaneous muscles and major fasciae of the ram.
Right lateral view. m = muscle, b = bone

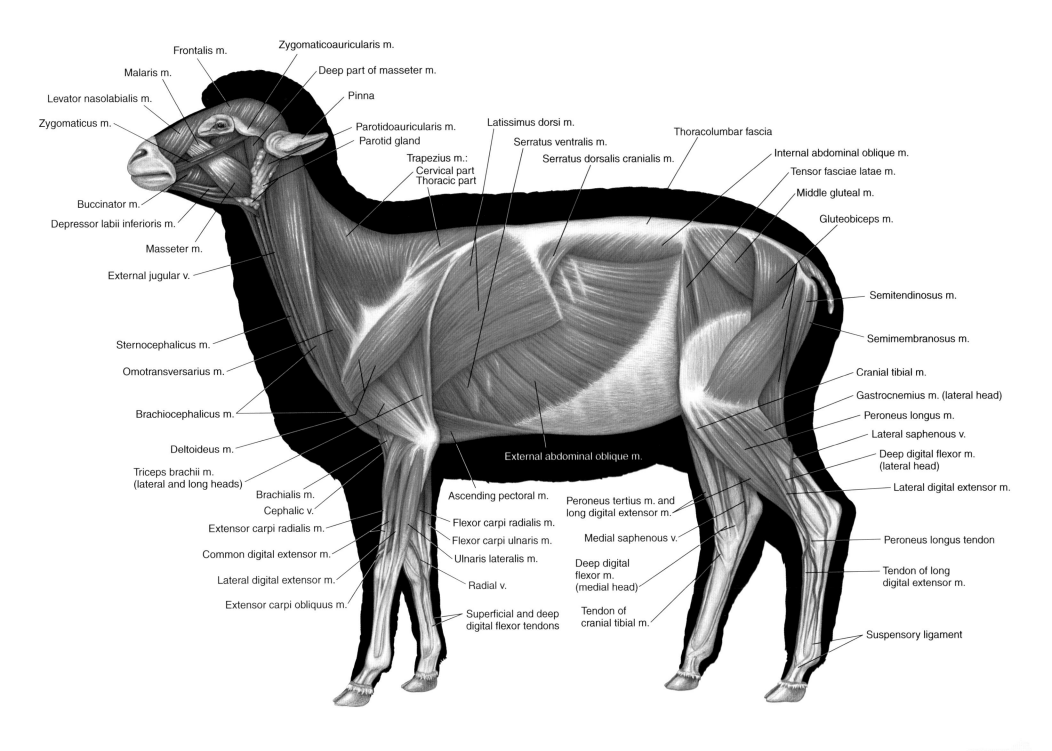

Frontalis m.

Zygomaticoauricularis m.

Malaris m.

Deep part of masseter m.

Levator nasolabialis m.

Pinna

Zygomaticus m.

Parotidoauricularis m.

Parotid gland

Latissimus dorsi m.

Thoracolumbar fascia

Serratus ventralis m.

Trapezius m.:
Cervical part
Thoracic part

Serratus dorsalis cranialis m.

Internal abdominal oblique m.

Tensor fasciae latae m.

Middle gluteal m.

Gluteobiceps m.

Buccinator m.

Depressor labii inferioris m.

Masseter m.

External jugular v.

Semitendinosus m.

Semimembranosus m.

Sternocephalicus m.

Omotransversarius m.

Cranial tibial m.

Gastrocnemius m. (lateral head)

Peroneus longus m.

Lateral saphenous v.

Brachiocephalicus m.

Deep digital flexor m.
(lateral head)

Deltoideus m.

Lateral digital extensor m.

Triceps brachii m.
(lateral and long heads)

Brachialis m.

Cephalic v.

Ascending pectoral m.

Peroneus tertius m. and
long digital extensor m.

Peroneus longus tendon

Extensor carpi radialis m.

Flexor carpi radialis m.

Medial saphenous v.

Common digital extensor m.

Flexor carpi ulnaris m.

Tendon of long
digital extensor m.

Lateral digital extensor m.

Ulnaris lateralis m.

Deep digital
flexor m.
(medial head)

Extensor carpi obliquus m.

Radial v.

External abdominal oblique m.

Superficial and deep
digital flexor tendons

Tendon of
cranial tibial m.

Suspensory ligament

**59**

**PLATE 3.6** Superficial muscles and veins of the ewe.  Left lateral view. m = muscle, v = vein

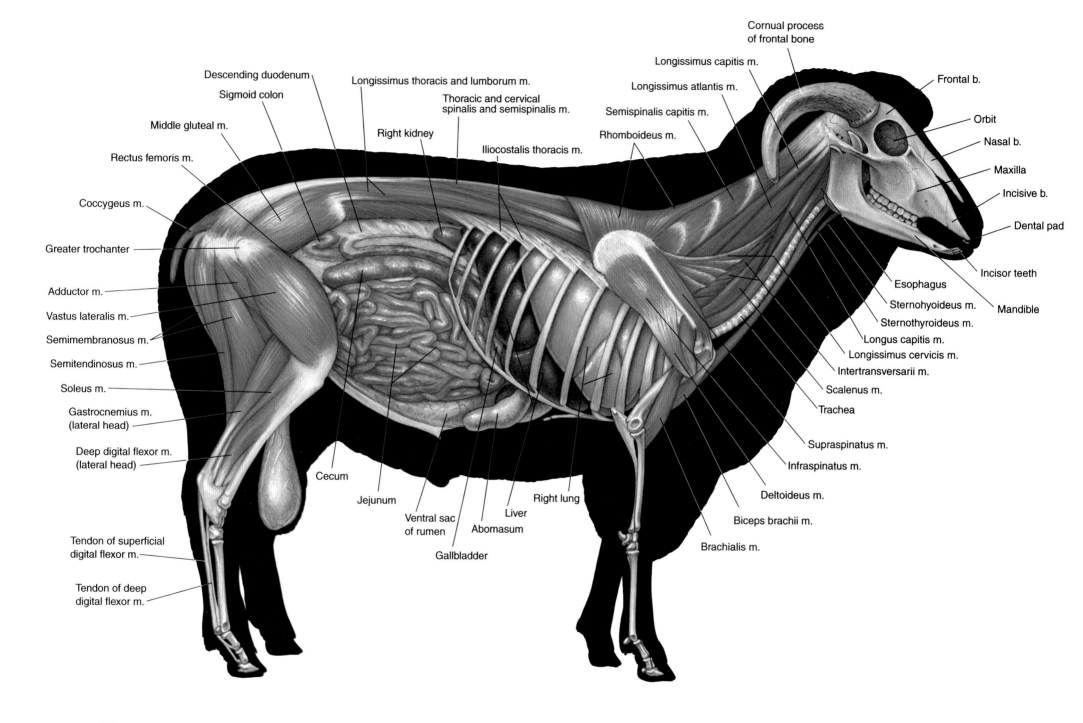

Descending duodenum

Sigmoid colon

Middle gluteal m.

Rectus femoris m.

Coccygeus m.

Greater trochanter

Adductor m.

Vastus lateralis m.

Semimembranosus m.

Semitendinosus m.

Soleus m.

Gastrocnemius m.
(lateral head)

Deep digital flexor m.
(lateral head)

Cecum

Jejunum

Ventral sac
of rumen

Gallbladder

Abomasum

Liver

Right lung

Tendon of superficial
digital flexor m.

Tendon of deep
digital flexor m.

Longissimus thoracis and lumborum m.

Thoracic and cervical
spinalis and semispinalis m.

Right kidney

Iliocostalis thoracis m.

Cornual process
of frontal bone

Longissimus capitis m.

Longissimus atlantis m.

Semispinalis capitis m.

Rhomboideus m.

Frontal b.

Orbit

Nasal b.

Maxilla

Incisive b.

Dental pad

Incisor teeth

Esophagus

Sternohyoideus m.

Mandible

Sternothyroideus m.

Longus capitis m.

Longissimus cervicis m.

Intertransversarii m.

Scalenus m.

Trachea

Supraspinatus m.

Infraspinatus m.

Deltoideus m.

Biceps brachii m.

Brachialis m.

**60**

**PLATE 3.7**  Deep cervical muscles and *in situ* viscera of the ram.  Omentum removed.
Right lateral view. m = muscle, b = bone

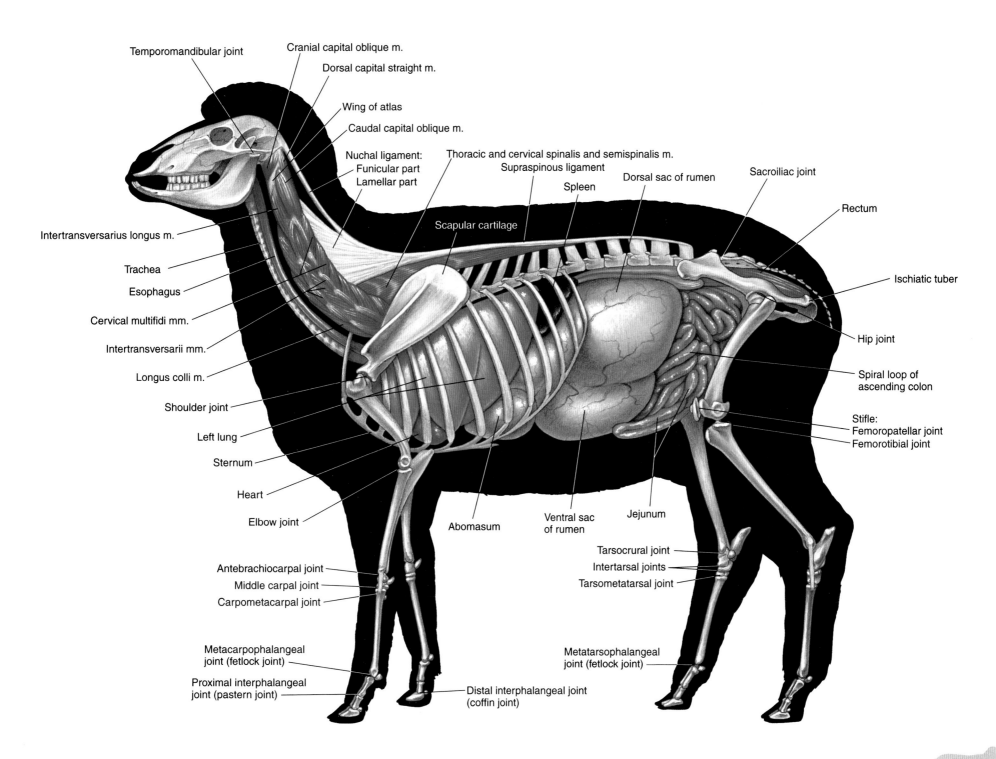

**PLATE 3.8**  Deep cervical muscles, *in situ* viscera, skeleton, and major joints of the ewe.  Left lateral view. m = muscle

61

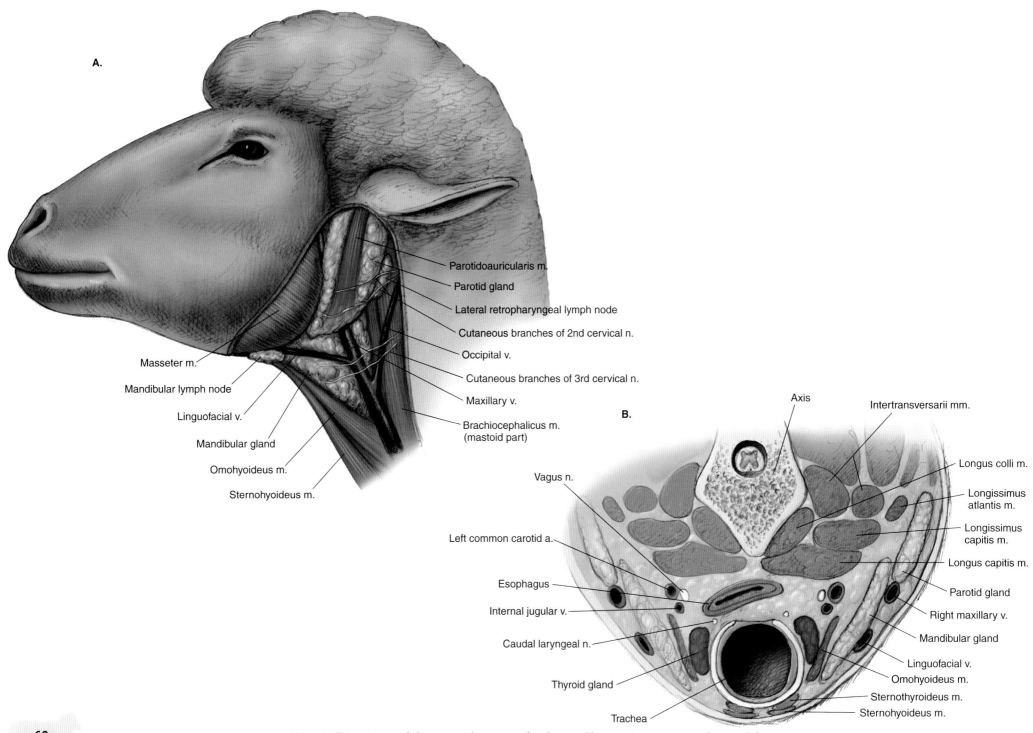

A.

Parotidoauricularis m.

Parotid gland

Lateral retropharyngeal lymph node

Cutaneous branches of 2nd cervical n.

Occipital v.

Cutaneous branches of 3rd cervical n.

Maxillary v.

Brachiocephalicus m.
(mastoid part)

Masseter m.

Mandibular lymph node

Linguofacial v.

Mandibular gland

Omohyoideus m.

Sternohyoideus m.

B.

Axis

Intertransversarii mm.

Longus colli m.

Longissimus
atlantis m.

Longissimus
capitis m.

Longus capitis m.

Parotid gland

Right maxillary v.

Mandibular gland

Linguofacial v.

Omohyoideus m.

Sternothyroideus m.

Sternohyoideus m.

Vagus n.

Left common carotid a.

Esophagus

Internal jugular v.

Caudal laryngeal n.

Thyroid gland

Trachea

62

**PLATE 3.9**  **A.** Dissection of the parotid region of a sheep.  Skin, cutaneous muscles, and fascia
are removed.  Left lateral view.  **B.** Cross-section of the neck at the level of the thyroid
gland.  Caudocranial view. m = muscle, v = vein, a = artery, n = nerve

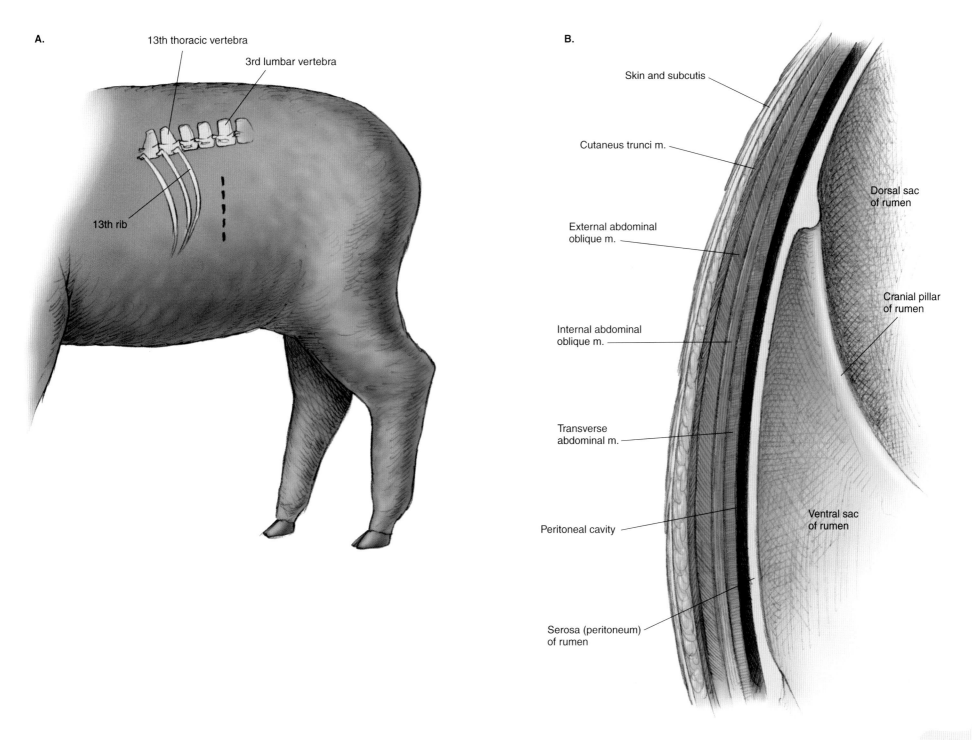

**A.** 13th thoracic vertebra

3rd lumbar vertebra

13th rib

**B.**

Skin and subcutis

Cutaneus trunci m.

External abdominal oblique m.

Internal abdominal oblique m.

Transverse abdominal m.

Peritoneal cavity

Serosa (peritoneum) of rumen

Dorsal sac of rumen

Cranial pillar of rumen

Ventral sac of rumen

63

**PLATE 3.10** **A.** Location of the left flank incision: *dashed line*. **B.** Cross-section through the left abdominal wall and subjacent ruminal wall. Caudocranial view. m = muscle

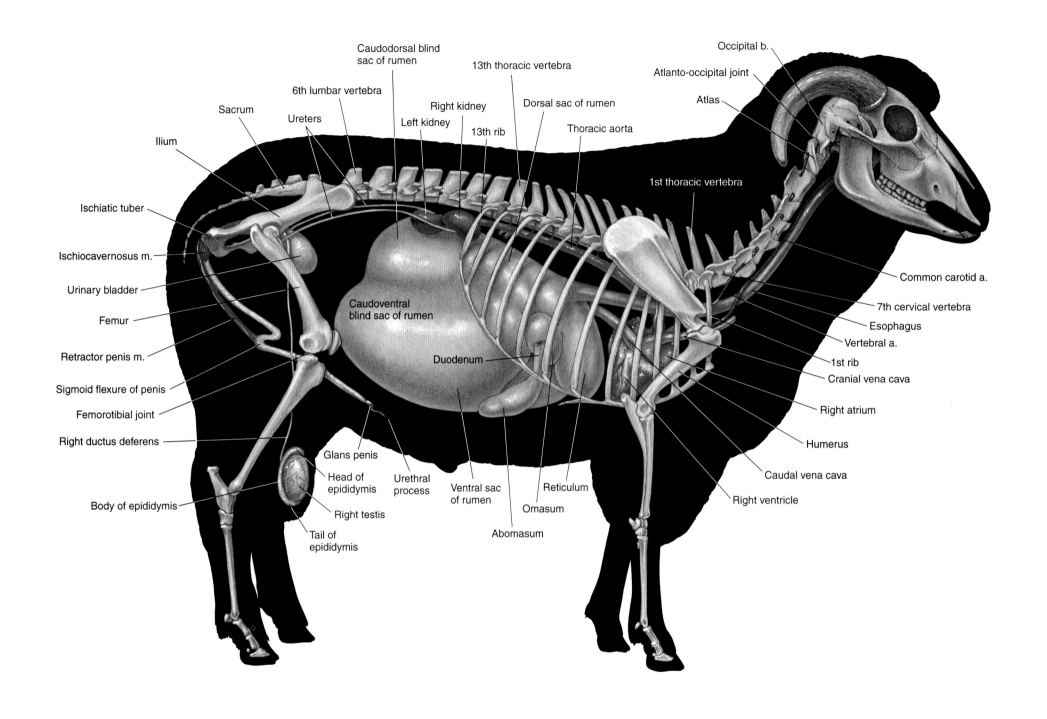

Caudodorsal blind sac of rumen

6th lumbar vertebra

13th thoracic vertebra

Occipital b.

Atlanto-occipital joint

Sacrum

Right kidney

Dorsal sac of rumen

Atlas

Ureters

Left kidney

13th rib

Thoracic aorta

Ilium

1st thoracic vertebra

Ischiatic tuber

Common carotid a.

Ischiocavernosus m.

7th cervical vertebra

Urinary bladder

Caudoventral
blind sac of rumen

Esophagus

Femur

Vertebral a.

Retractor penis m.

Duodenum

1st rib

Cranial vena cava

Sigmoid flexure of penis

Femorotibial joint

Right atrium

Right ductus deferens

Humerus

Glans penis

Head of
epididymis

Urethral
process

Ventral sac
of rumen

Reticulum

Caudal vena cava

Body of epididymis

Right testis

Omasum

Right ventricle

Tail of
epididymis

Abomasum

**PLATE 3.11** Reproductive organs, urinary organs, esophagus and stomach, heart, and
adjacent major vessels related to the skeleton of the ram. Right lateral view.
b = bone, m = muscle, a = artery

64

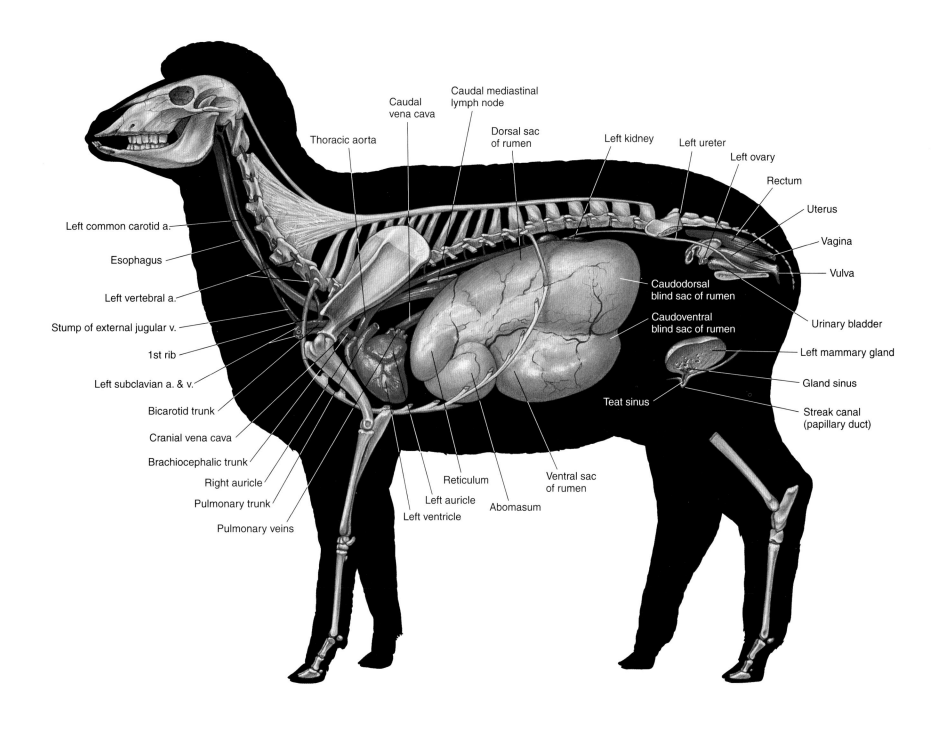

Left common carotid a.

Esophagus

Left vertebral a.

Stump of external jugular v.

1st rib

Left subclavian a. & v.

Bicarotid trunk

Cranial vena cava

Brachiocephalic trunk

Right auricle

Pulmonary trunk

Pulmonary veins

Thoracic aorta

Caudal vena cava

Caudal mediastinal lymph node

Dorsal sac of rumen

Left kidney

Left ureter

Left ovary

Rectum

Uterus

Vagina

Vulva

Caudodorsal blind sac of rumen

Caudoventral blind sac of rumen

Urinary bladder

Left mammary gland

Gland sinus

Teat sinus

Streak canal (papillary duct)

Reticulum

Left auricle

Left ventricle

Abomasum

Ventral sac of rumen

**PLATE 3.12** Reproductive organs, urinary organs, heart, and adjacent major vessels, esophagus and stomach of the ewe. Left lateral view. a = artery, v = vein

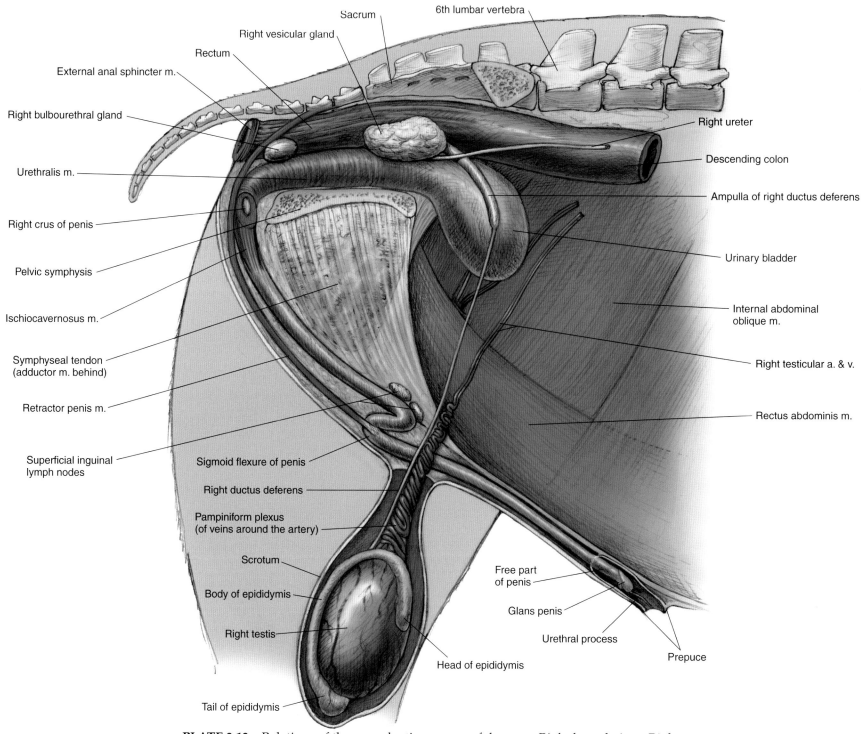

Sacrum

6th lumbar vertebra

Right vesicular gland

Rectum

External anal sphincter m.

Right bulbourethral gland

Right ureter

Urethralis m.

Descending colon

Ampulla of right ductus deferens

Right crus of penis

Pelvic symphysis

Urinary bladder

Ischiocavernosus m.

Internal abdominal oblique m.

Symphyseal tendon (adductor m. behind)

Right testicular a. & v.

Retractor penis m.

Rectus abdominis m.

Superficial inguinal lymph nodes

Sigmoid flexure of penis

Right ductus deferens

Pampiniform plexus (of veins around the artery)

Scrotum

Free part of penis

Body of epididymis

Glans penis

Right testis

Urethral process

Prepuce

Head of epididymis

Tail of epididymis

**PLATE 3.13** Relations of the reproductive organs of the ram. Right lateral view. Right pelvic limb and body wall are removed. The ram's prostate gland is entirely disseminate; it lies deep to the urethralis muscle. m = muscle, a = artery, v = vein

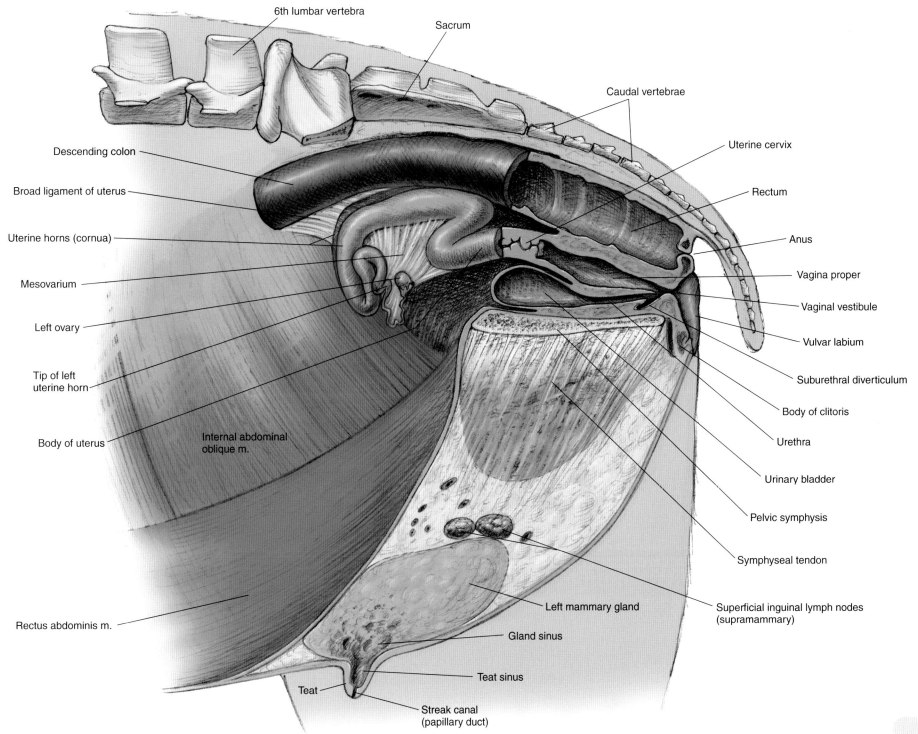

6th lumbar vertebra

Sacrum

Caudal vertebrae

Descending colon

Uterine cervix

Broad ligament of uterus

Rectum

Uterine horns (cornua)

Anus

Mesovarium

Vagina proper

Left ovary

Vaginal vestibule

Vulvar labium

Tip of left
uterine horn

Suburethral diverticulum

Body of uterus

Internal abdominal
oblique m.

Body of clitoris

Urethra

Urinary bladder

Pelvic symphysis

Rectus abdominis m.

Symphyseal tendon

Left mammary gland

Superficial inguinal lymph nodes
(supramammary)

Gland sinus

Teat sinus

Teat

Streak canal
(papillary duct)

**PLATE 3.14** Relations of the reproductive organs of the ewe. Left lateral view with partial
median sections of the vagina, uterine cervix, rectum, urinary bladder, and urethra. m = muscle

67

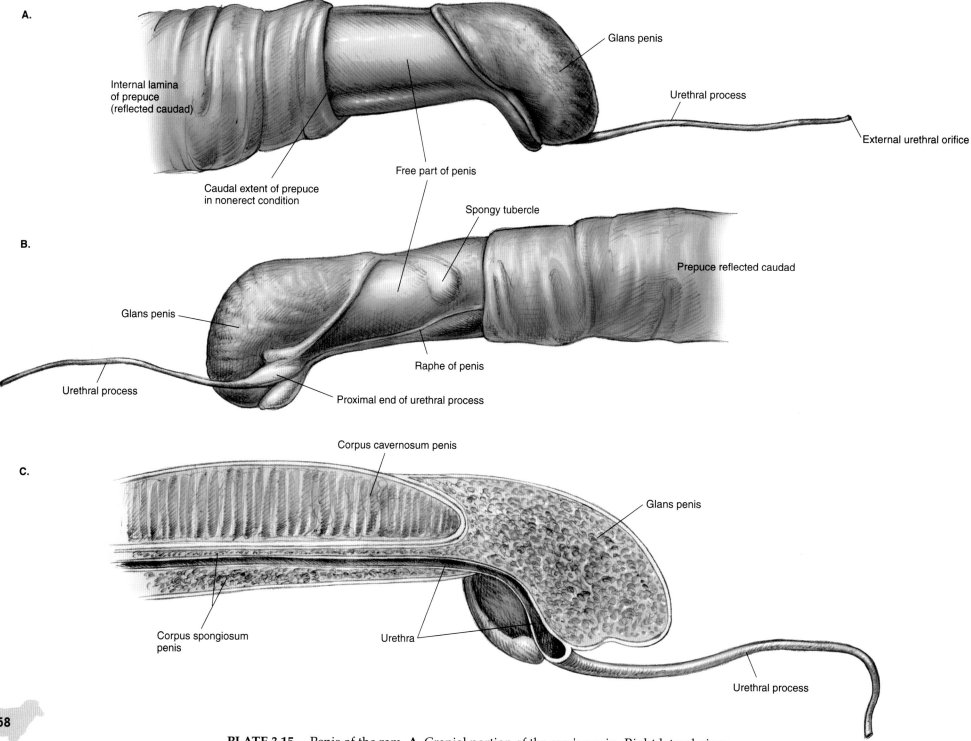

A.

Glans penis

Urethral process

Internal lamina
of prepuce
(reflected caudad)

External urethral orifice

Free part of penis

Caudal extent of prepuce
in nonerect condition

Spongy tubercle

B.

Prepuce reflected caudad

Glans penis

Raphe of penis

Urethral process

Proximal end of urethral process

Corpus cavernosum penis

C.

Glans penis

Corpus spongiosum
penis

Urethra

Urethral process

68

**PLATE 3.15**   Penis of the ram. **A.** Cranial portion of the ram's penis.  Right lateral view.
**B.** Left lateral view.  **C.** Median section.  Right lateral view.

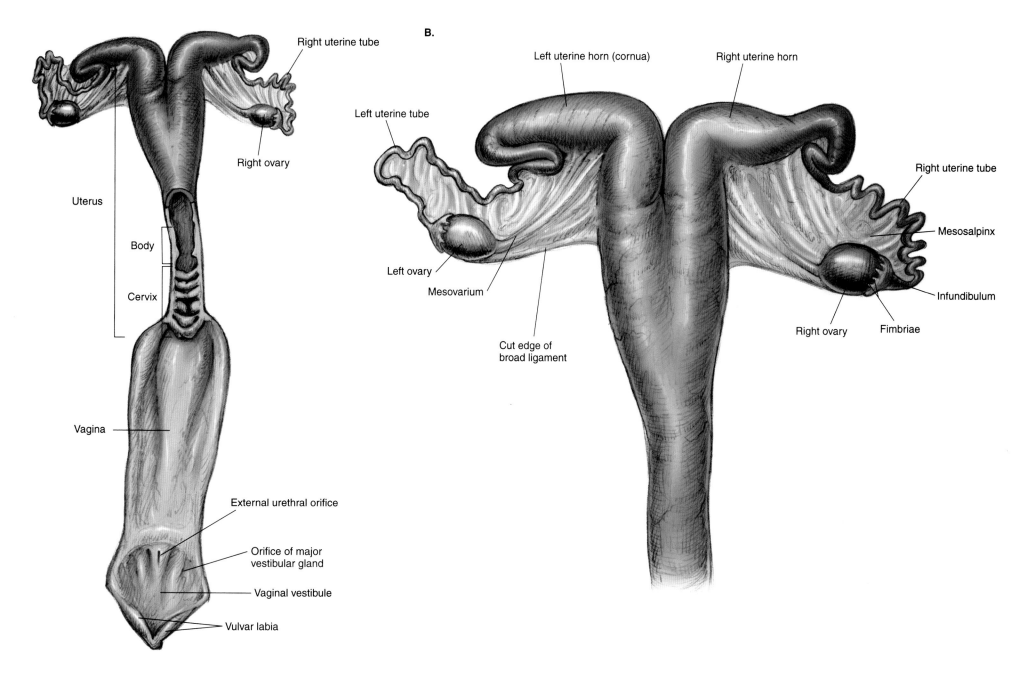

**A.**

Right uterine tube

Right ovary

Uterus

Body

Cervix

Vagina

External urethral orifice

Orifice of major vestibular gland

Vaginal vestibule

Vulvar labia

**B.**

Left uterine tube

Left uterine horn (cornua)

Right uterine horn

Right uterine tube

Mesosalpinx

Left ovary

Mesovarium

Cut edge of broad ligament

Right ovary

Fimbriae

Infundibulum

**PLATE 3.16** **A.** Isolated reproductive organs of the ewe. Vagina and a portion of the uterus opened dorsally. **B.** Isolated uterus, uterine tubes, and ovaries of the ewe. Dorsal view.

69

# SECTION 4  THE GOAT (*Capra hircus*)

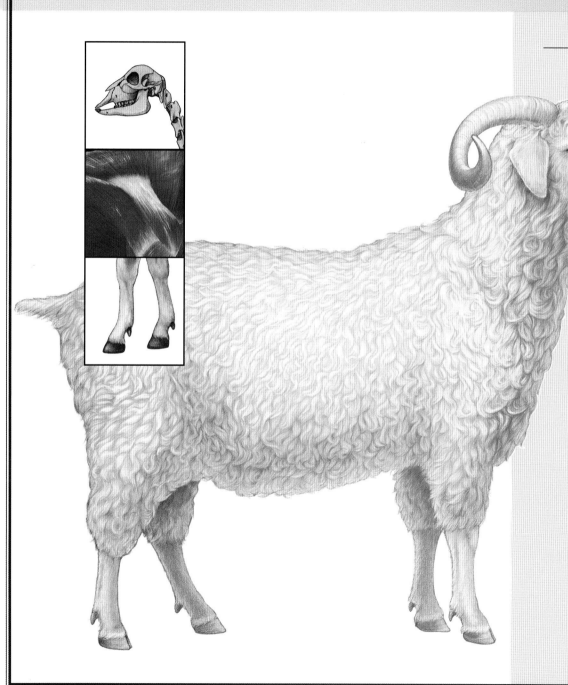

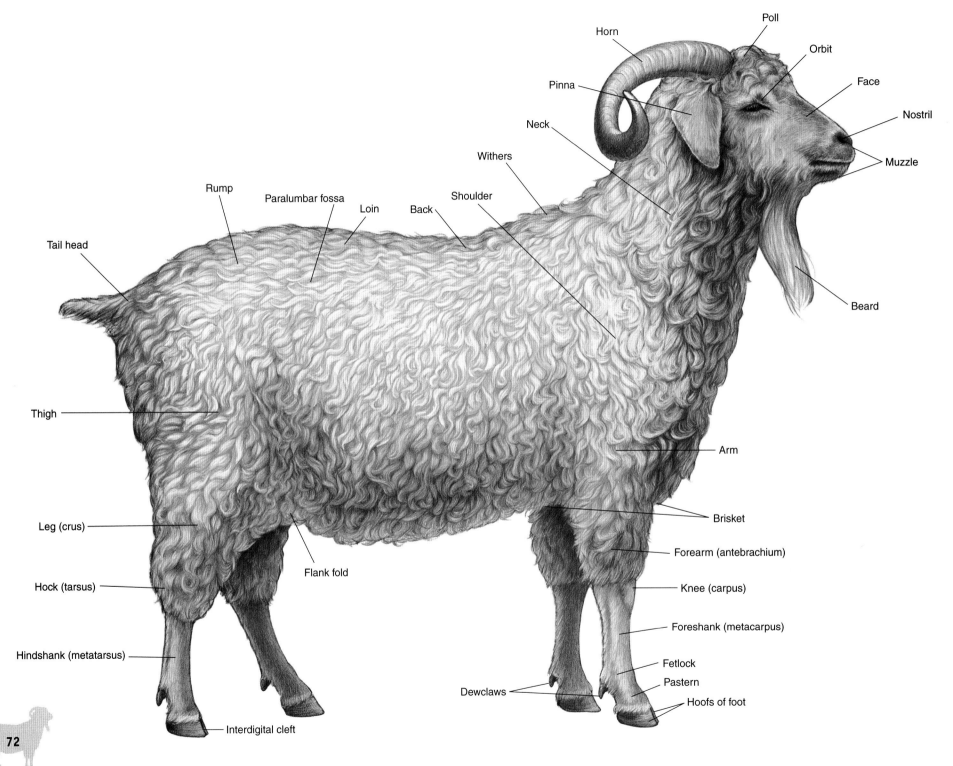

Horn

Poll

Orbit

Pinna

Face

Neck

Nostril

Withers

Muzzle

Rump

Paralumbar fossa

Shoulder

Loin

Back

Tail head

Beard

Thigh

Arm

Leg (crus)

Brisket

Forearm (antebrachium)

Hock (tarsus)

Flank fold

Knee (carpus)

Foreshank (metacarpus)

Hindshank (metatarsus)

Fetlock

Pastern

Dewclaws

Hoofs of foot

72

Interdigital cleft

**PLATE 4.1** Right lateral view of an Angora buck (billy).

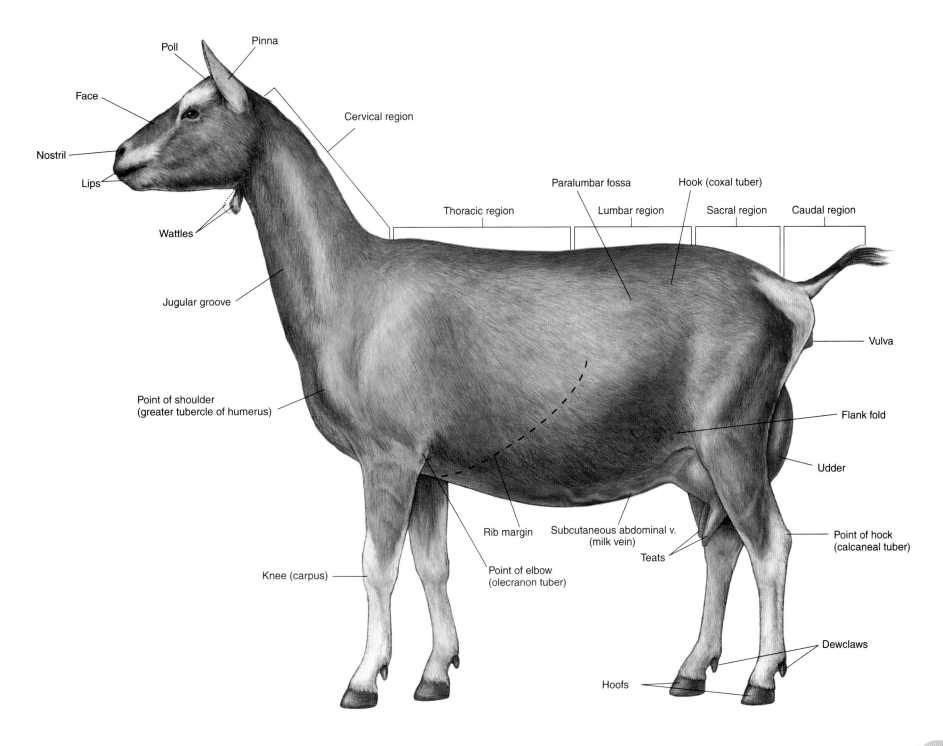

**PLATE 4.2** Left lateral view of a Toggenberg doe (nanny).
Dorsal vertebral regions are indicated. v = vein

73

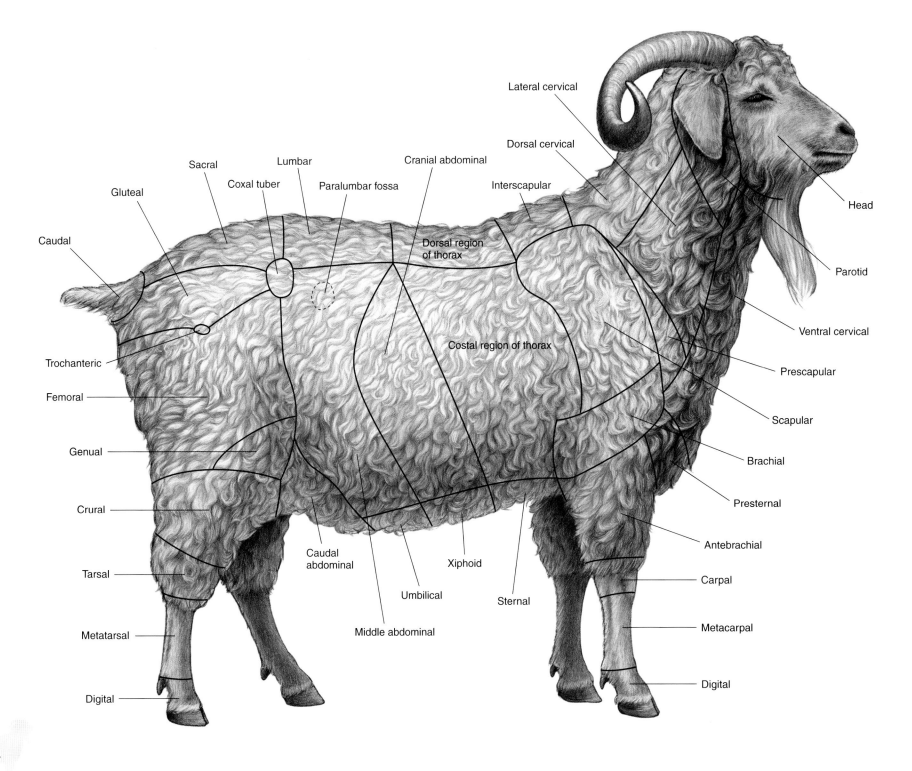

74

**PLATE 4.3**   Body regions of the goat.   Right lateral view.

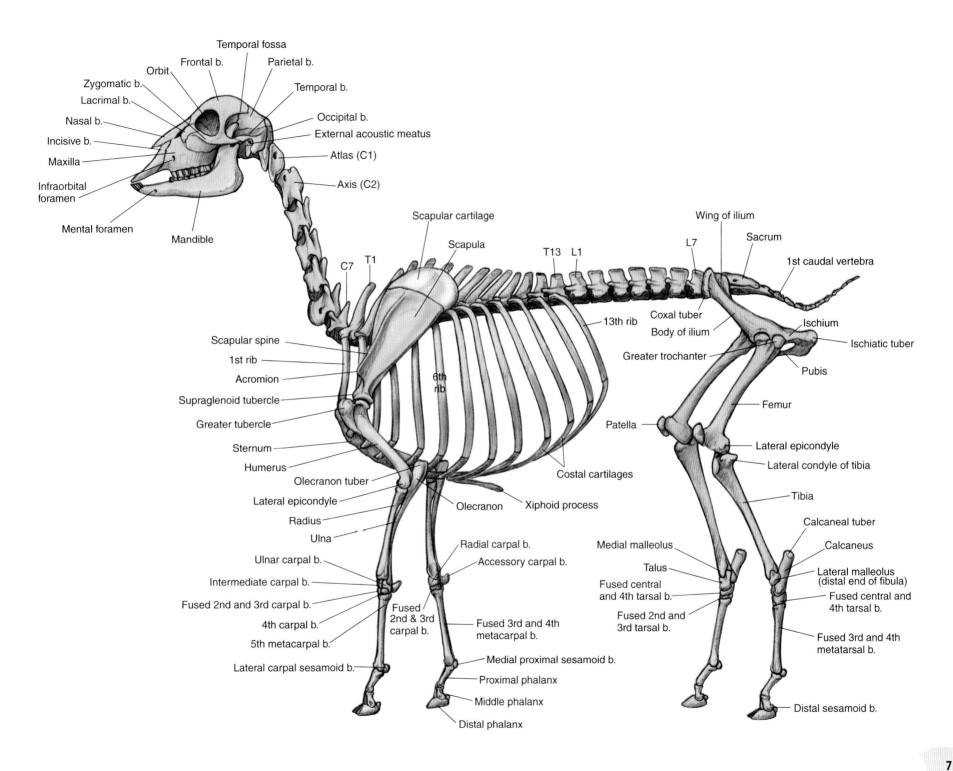

Temporal fossa

Frontal b.

Parietal b.

Orbit

Temporal b.

Zygomatic b.

Lacrimal b.

Occipital b.

Nasal b.

External acoustic meatus

Incisive b.

Atlas (C1)

Maxilla

Axis (C2)

Infraorbital foramen

Mental foramen

Mandible

Scapular cartilage

Wing of ilium

Scapula

Sacrum

L7

T13  L1

1st caudal vertebra

C7  T1

Coxal tuber

13th rib

Body of ilium

Ischium

Scapular spine

Greater trochanter

Ischiatic tuber

1st rib

Pubis

Acromion

Supraglenoid tubercle

Greater tubercle

Femur

Sternum

Patella

Humerus

Lateral epicondyle

Olecranon tuber

Lateral condyle of tibia

Lateral epicondyle

Costal cartilages

Radius

Olecranon

Xiphoid process

Tibia

Ulna

Radial carpal b.

Medial malleolus

Calcaneal tuber

Accessory carpal b.

Ulnar carpal b.

Talus

Calcaneus

Intermediate carpal b.

Fused central and 4th tarsal b.

Lateral malleolus (distal end of fibula)

Fused 2nd and 3rd carpal b.

Fused 2nd & 3rd carpal b.

Fused central and 4th tarsal b.

4th carpal b.

Fused 3rd and 4th metacarpal b.

Fused 2nd and 3rd tarsal b.

5th metacarpal b.

Fused 3rd and 4th metatarsal b.

Lateral carpal sesamoid b.

Medial proximal sesamoid b.

Proximal phalanx

Middle phalanx

Distal sesamoid b.

Distal phalanx

6th rib

**75**

**PLATE 4.4**  Skeleton of the goat.  Left lateral view. b = bone, C = cervical vertebra, T = thoracic vertebra, L = lumbar vertebra

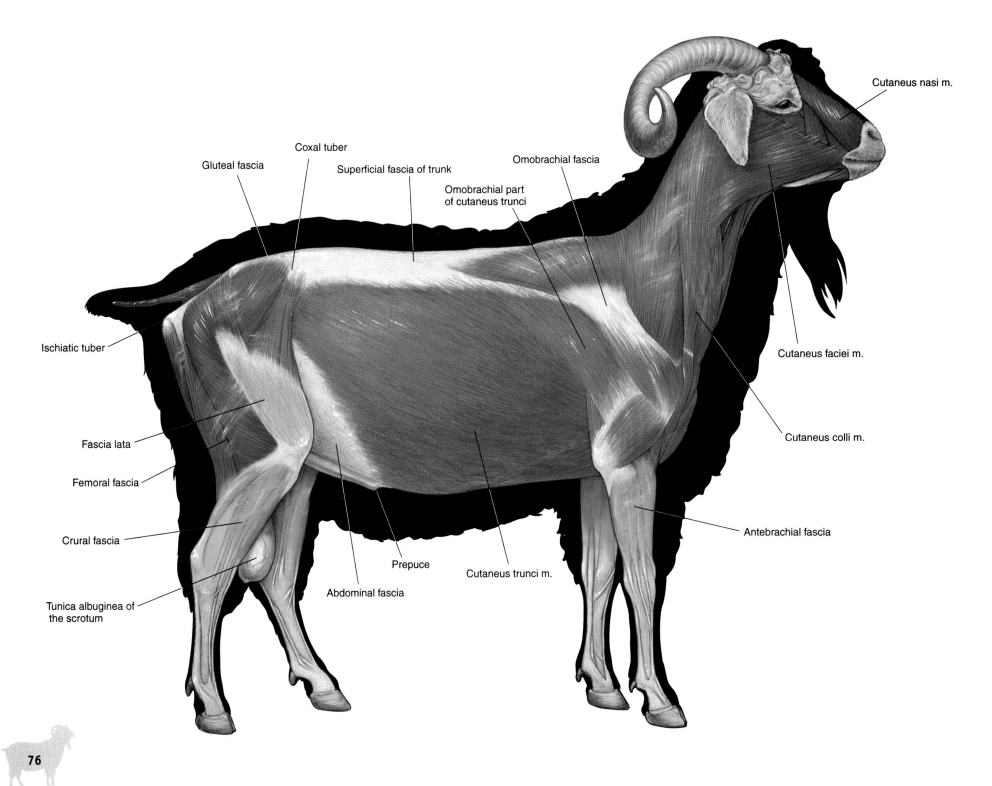

Gluteal fascia

Coxal tuber

Superficial fascia of trunk

Omobrachial fascia

Omobrachial part
of cutaneus trunci

Cutaneus nasi m.

Ischiatic tuber

Cutaneus faciei m.

Fascia lata

Cutaneus colli m.

Femoral fascia

Crural fascia

Antebrachial fascia

Prepuce

Cutaneus trunci m.

Abdominal fascia

Tunica albuginea of
the scrotum

76

**PLATE 4.5**  Cutaneous muscles and major fasciae of the buck.  Right lateral view. m = muscle

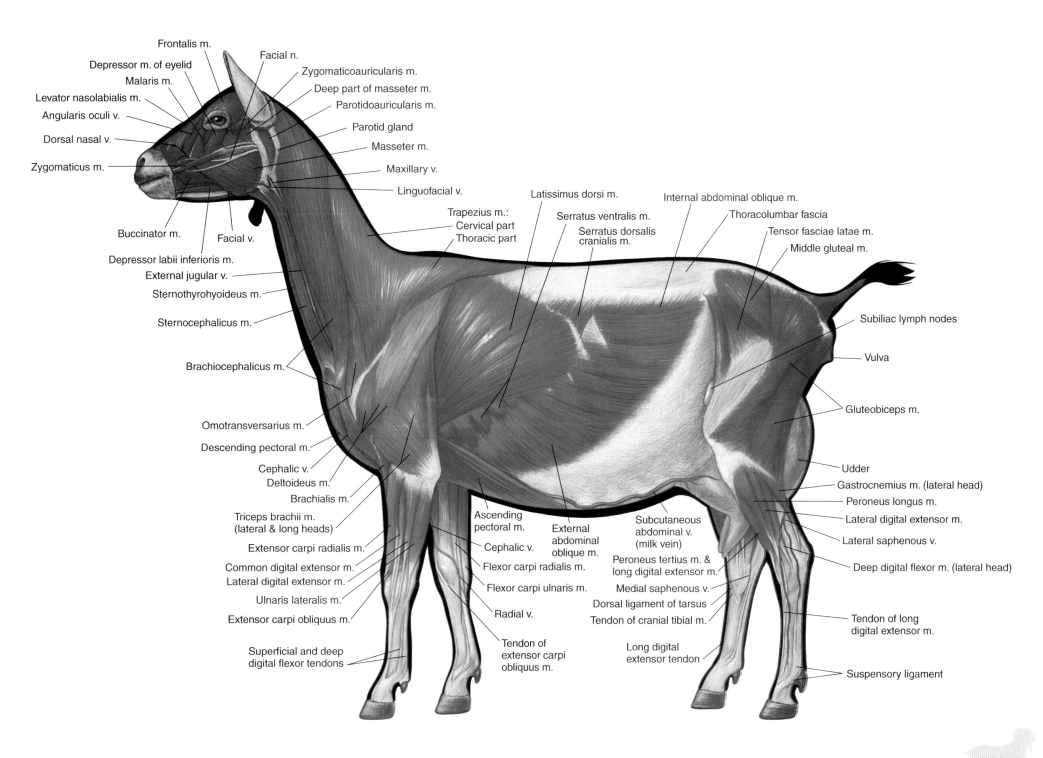

Frontalis m.
Depressor m. of eyelid
Malaris m.
Levator nasolabialis m.
Angularis oculi v.
Dorsal nasal v.
Zygomaticus m.
Buccinator m.
Facial v.
Depressor labii inferioris m.
External jugular v.
Sternothyrohyoideus m.
Sternocephalicus m.
Brachiocephalicus m.
Omotransversarius m.
Descending pectoral m.
Cephalic v.
Deltoideus m.
Brachialis m.
Triceps brachii m. (lateral & long heads)
Extensor carpi radialis m.
Common digital extensor m.
Lateral digital extensor m.
Ulnaris lateralis m.
Extensor carpi obliquus m.
Superficial and deep digital flexor tendons

Facial n.
Zygomaticoauricularis m.
Deep part of masseter m.
Parotidoauricularis m.
Parotid gland
Masseter m.
Maxillary v.
Linguofacial v.
Trapezius m.:
Cervical part
Thoracic part

Latissimus dorsi m.
Serratus ventralis m.
Serratus dorsalis cranialis m.

Internal abdominal oblique m.
Thoracolumbar fascia
Tensor fasciae latae m.
Middle gluteal m.

Subiliac lymph nodes
Vulva
Gluteobiceps m.
Udder
Gastrocnemius m. (lateral head)
Peroneus longus m.
Lateral digital extensor m.
Lateral saphenous v.
Deep digital flexor m. (lateral head)
Tendon of long digital extensor m.
Suspensory ligament

Ascending pectoral m.
Cephalic v.
Flexor carpi radialis m.
Flexor carpi ulnaris m.
Radial v.
Tendon of extensor carpi obliquus m.

External abdominal oblique m.
Subcutaneous abdominal v. (milk vein)
Peroneus tertius m. & long digital extensor m.
Medial saphenous v.
Dorsal ligament of tarsus
Tendon of cranial tibial m.
Long digital extensor tendon

77

**PLATE 4.6** Superficial muscles and veins of the doe. Left lateral view. m = muscle, v = vein

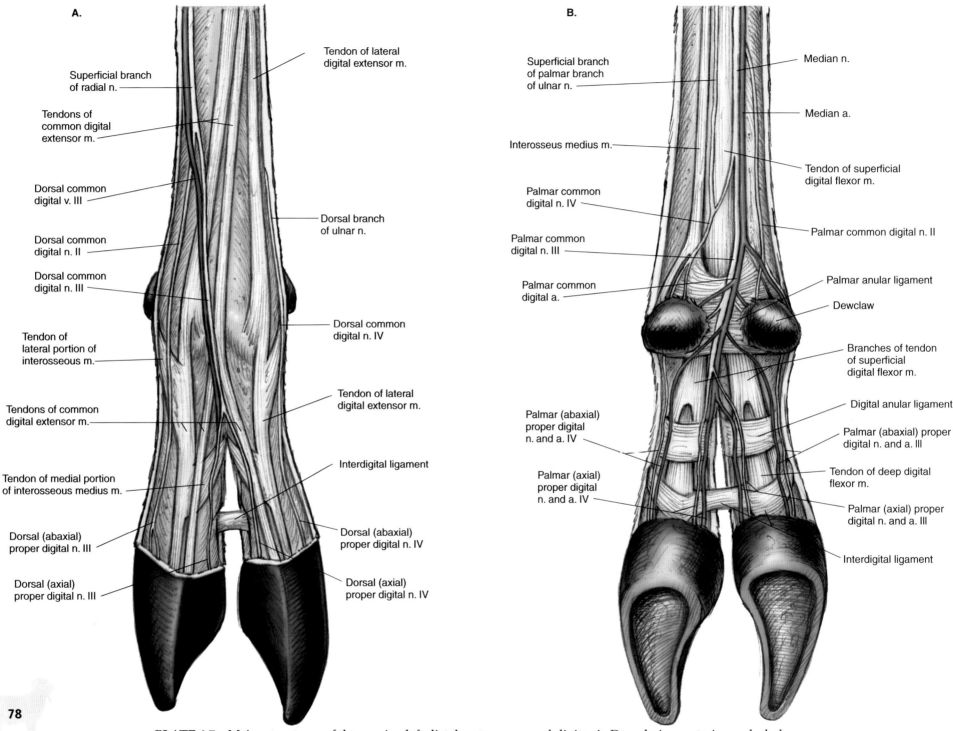

**A.**

Superficial branch of radial n.

Tendons of common digital extensor m.

Dorsal common digital v. III

Dorsal common digital n. II

Dorsal common digital n. III

Tendon of lateral portion of interosseous m.

Tendons of common digital extensor m.

Tendon of medial portion of interosseous medius m.

Dorsal (abaxial) proper digital n. III

Dorsal (axial) proper digital n. III

Tendon of lateral digital extensor m.

Dorsal branch of ulnar n.

Dorsal common digital n. IV

Tendon of lateral digital extensor m.

Interdigital ligament

Dorsal (abaxial) proper digital n. IV

Dorsal (axial) proper digital n. IV

**B.**

Superficial branch of palmar branch of ulnar n.

Interosseus medius m.

Palmar common digital n. IV

Palmar common digital n. III

Palmar common digital a.

Palmar (abaxial) proper digital n. and a. IV

Palmar (axial) proper digital n. and a. IV

Median n.

Median a.

Tendon of superficial digital flexor m.

Palmar common digital n. II

Palmar anular ligament

Dewclaw

Branches of tendon of superficial digital flexor m.

Digital anular ligament

Palmar (abaxial) proper digital n. and a. III

Tendon of deep digital flexor m.

Palmar (axial) proper digital n. and a. III

Interdigital ligament

78

**PLATE 4.7**  Major structures of the caprine left distal metacarpus and digits. **A.** Dorsal view, arteries excluded.
**B.** Palmar view, veins excluded. n = nerve, m = muscle, a = artery

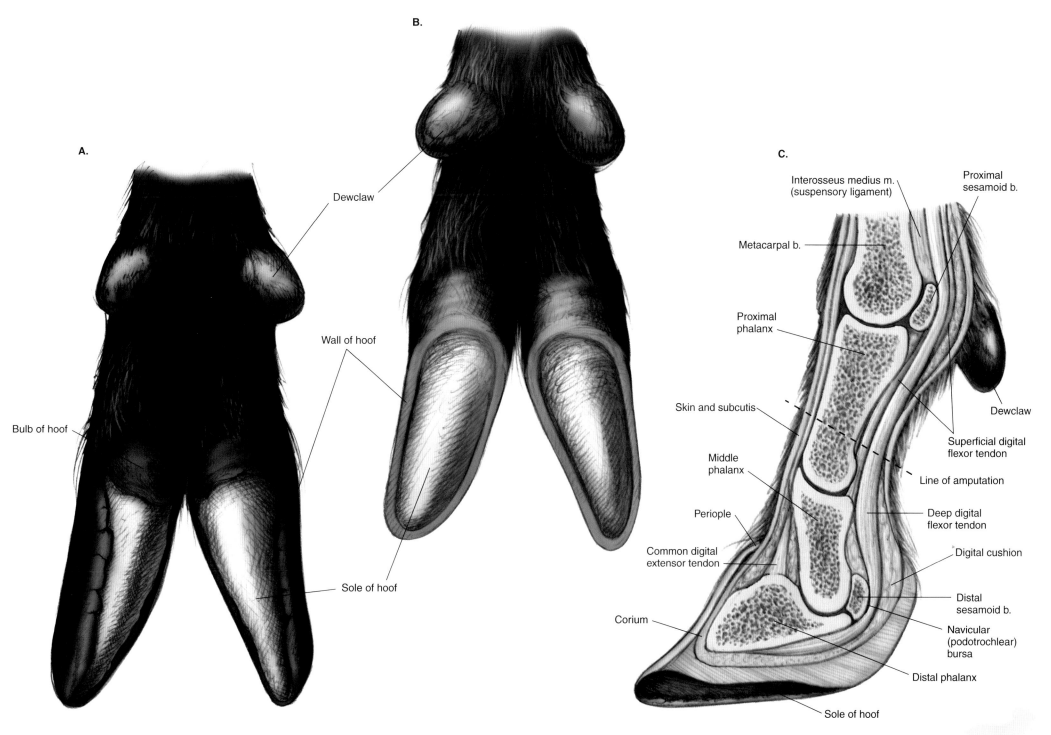

**PLATE 4.8** **A.** Untrimmed hoofs of the goat. **B.** Trimmed hoofs of the goat. **C.** Parasagittal section through the fetlock and digit. For artiodactyls, claw is synonymous with hoof. When kept on soft ground, a mature goat's hoofs should be trimmed every 4–5 months. b = bone

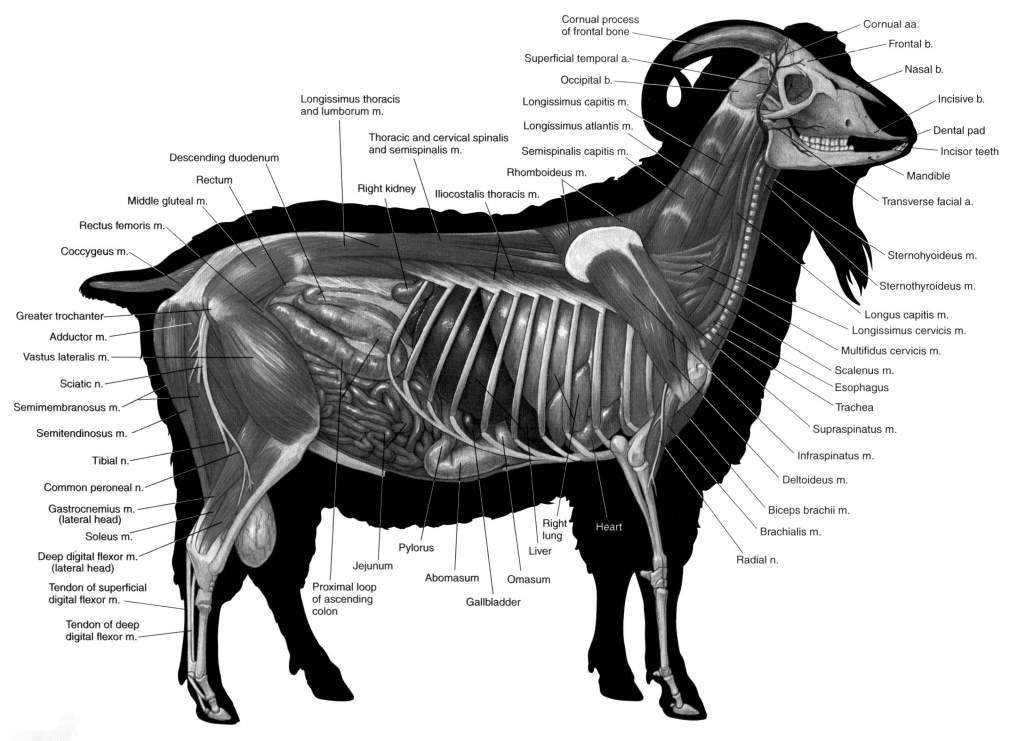

Cornual process of frontal bone

Superficial temporal a.

Occipital b.

Cornual aa.

Frontal b.

Nasal b.

Incisive b.

Dental pad

Incisor teeth

Mandible

Transverse facial a.

Longissimus capitis m.

Longissimus atlantis m.

Semispinalis capitis m.

Rhomboideus m.

Iliocostalis thoracis m.

Longissimus thoracis and lumborum m.

Thoracic and cervical spinalis and semispinalis m.

Right kidney

Descending duodenum

Rectum

Middle gluteal m.

Rectus femoris m.

Coccygeus m.

Greater trochanter

Adductor m.

Vastus lateralis m.

Sciatic n.

Semimembranosus m.

Semitendinosus m.

Tibial n.

Common peroneal n.

Gastrocnemius m. (lateral head)

Soleus m.

Deep digital flexor m. (lateral head)

Tendon of superficial digital flexor m.

Tendon of deep digital flexor m.

Sternohyoideus m.

Sternothyroideus m.

Longus capitis m.

Longissimus cervicis m.

Multifidus cervicis m.

Scalenus m.

Esophagus

Trachea

Supraspinatus m.

Infraspinatus m.

Deltoideus m.

Biceps brachii m.

Brachialis m.

Radial n.

Heart

Right lung

Liver

Omasum

Gallbladder

Abomasum

Pylorus

Jejunum

Proximal loop of ascending colon

80

**PLATE 4.9** Deep muscles and *in situ* viscera of the buck. Greater omentum is removed. Right lateral view. m = muscle, n = nerve, a = artery, b = bone

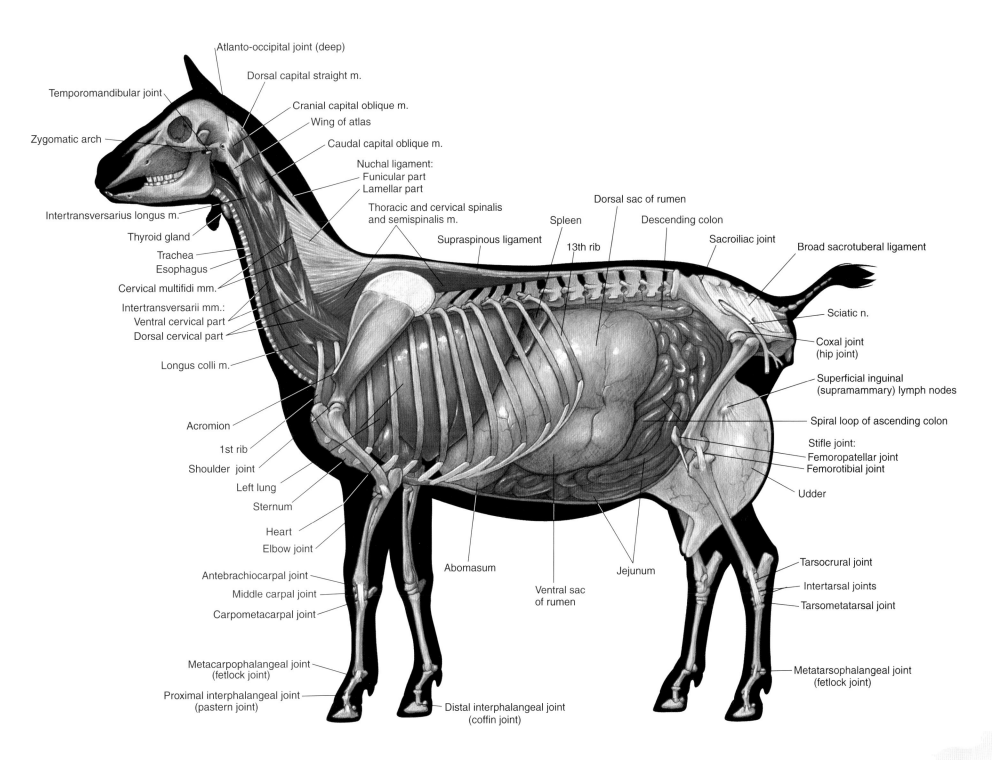

**PLATE 4.10** Deep cervical muscles, *in situ* viscera, skeleton, and major joints of the doe.
Left lateral view. m = muscle, n = nerve

81

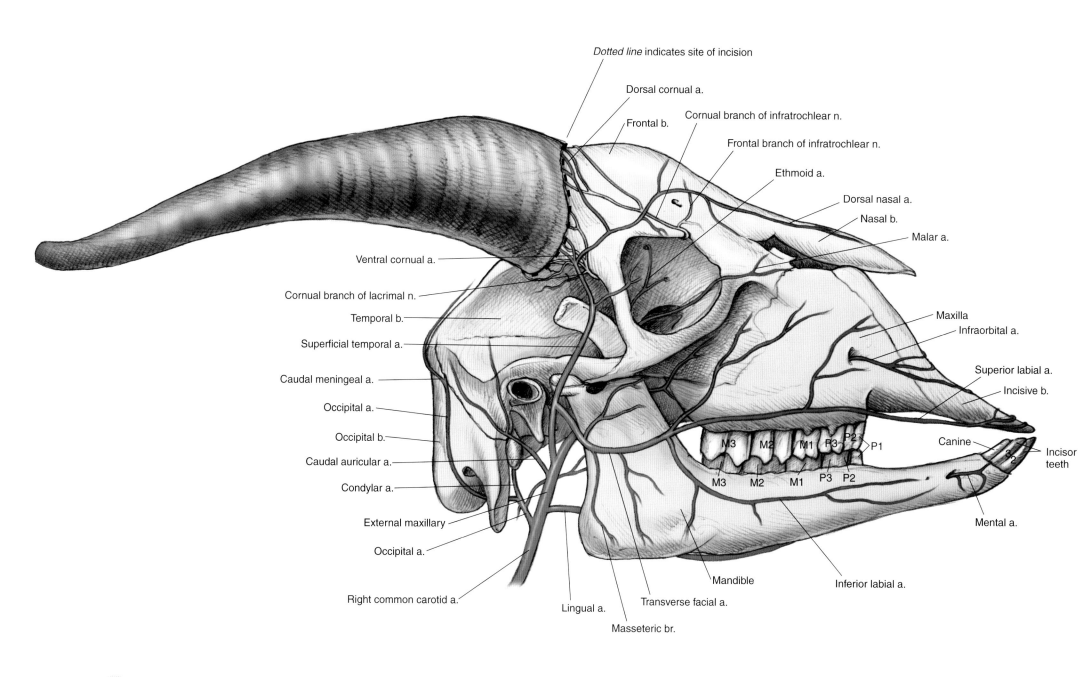

Dotted line indicates site of incision

Dorsal cornual a.

Cornual branch of infratrochlear n.

Frontal b.

Frontal branch of infratrochlear n.

Ethmoid a.

Dorsal nasal a.

Nasal b.

Malar a.

Ventral cornual a.

Cornual branch of lacrimal n.

Maxilla

Temporal b.

Infraorbital a.

Superficial temporal a.

Caudal meningeal a.

Superior labial a.

Incisive b.

Occipital a.

M3   M2   M1   P3   P2   P1

Canine

Occipital b.

Incisor teeth

Caudal auricular a.

M3    M2    M1    P3   P2

Condylar a.

External maxillary

Mental a.

Occipital a.

Right common carotid a.

Mandible

Inferior labial a.

Lingual a.

Transverse facial a.

Masseteric br.

**PLATE 4.11**   Superficial structures of the goat's head.  *Dashed line* indicates the site of a dehorning incision.
a = artery, b = bone, n = nerve, M = molar tooth, P = premolar tooth

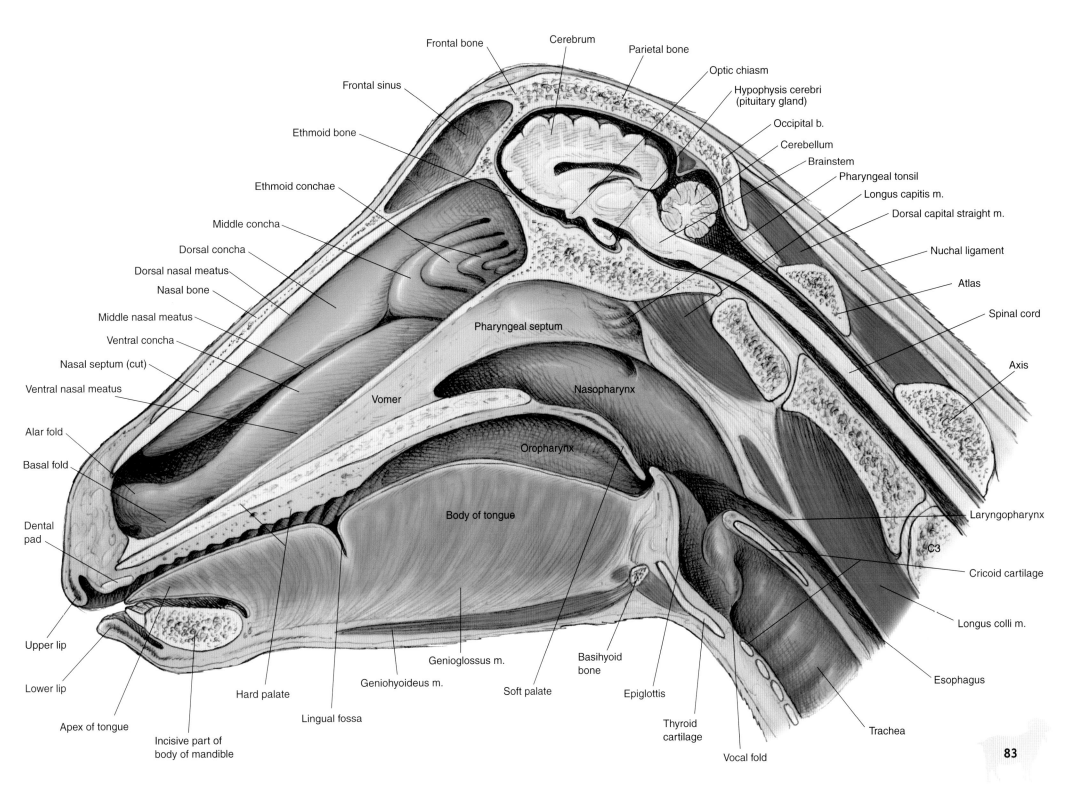

**PLATE 4.12**  Median section of the caprine head. Most of the nasal septum is removed. m = muscle, b = bone

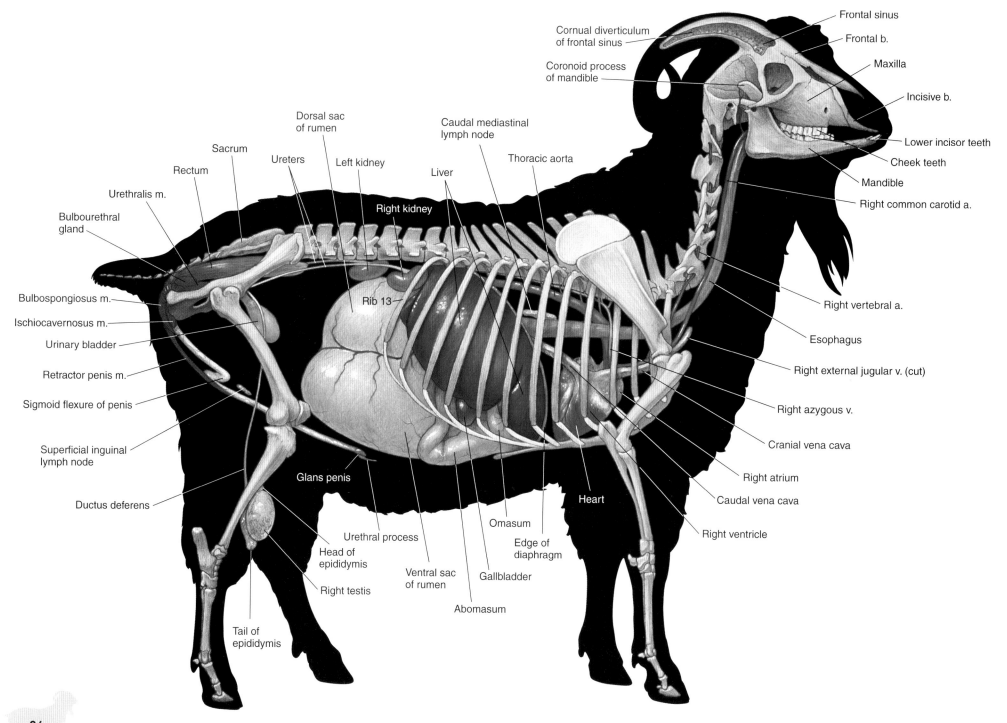

Cornual diverticulum of frontal sinus

Coronoid process of mandible

Frontal sinus

Frontal b.

Maxilla

Incisive b.

Lower incisor teeth

Cheek teeth

Mandible

Right common carotid a.

Right vertebral a.

Esophagus

Right external jugular v. (cut)

Right azygous v.

Cranial vena cava

Right atrium

Caudal vena cava

Right ventricle

Dorsal sac of rumen

Caudal mediastinal lymph node

Sacrum

Ureters

Left kidney

Liver

Thoracic aorta

Rectum

Urethralis m.

Right kidney

Bulbourethral gland

Bulbospongiosus m.

Rib 13

Ischiocavernosus m.

Urinary bladder

Retractor penis m.

Sigmoid flexure of penis

Superficial inguinal lymph node

Ductus deferens

Glans penis

Urethral process

Head of epididymis

Right testis

Ventral sac of rumen

Gallbladder

Omasum

Edge of diaphragm

Heart

Abomasum

Tail of epididymis

**PLATE 4.13**   Reproductive organs, abdominal viscera, heart, and adjacent major vessels related to the skeleton of the buck. Intestines and lungs removed. Right lateral view.
m = muscle, v = vein, a = artery, b = bone

84

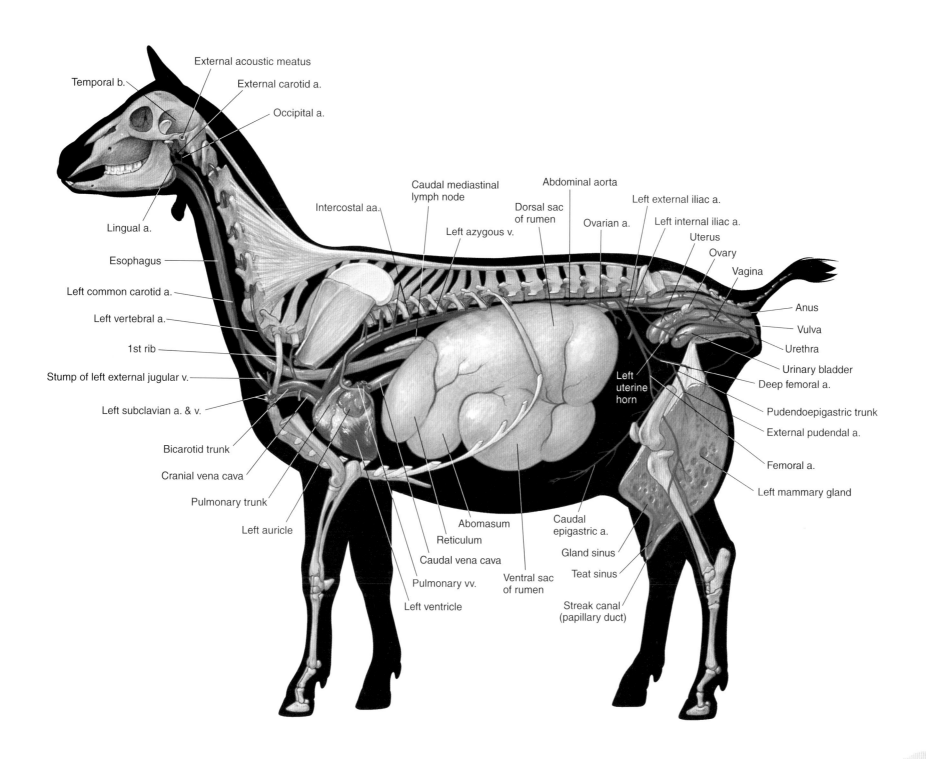

Temporal b.

External acoustic meatus

External carotid a.

Occipital a.

Lingual a.

Esophagus

Left common carotid a.

Left vertebral a.

1st rib

Stump of left external jugular v.

Left subclavian a. & v.

Bicarotid trunk

Cranial vena cava

Pulmonary trunk

Left auricle

Intercostal aa.

Caudal mediastinal
lymph node

Left azygous v.

Abdominal aorta

Dorsal sac
of rumen

Ovarian a.

Left external iliac a.

Left internal iliac a.

Uterus

Ovary

Vagina

Anus

Vulva

Urethra

Urinary bladder

Deep femoral a.

Left
uterine
horn

Pudendoepigastric trunk

External pudendal a.

Femoral a.

Left mammary gland

Abomasum

Reticulum

Caudal vena cava

Left ventricle

Pulmonary vv.

Caudal
epigastric a.

Gland sinus

Teat sinus

Ventral sac
of rumen

Streak canal
(papillary duct)

**PLATE 4.14** Reproductive organs, abdominal viscera, heart, and adjacent major
vessels of the doe. Ribs 2 and 12 and the lungs and intestines are removed.
Left lateral view. a = artery, b = bone, v = vein

85

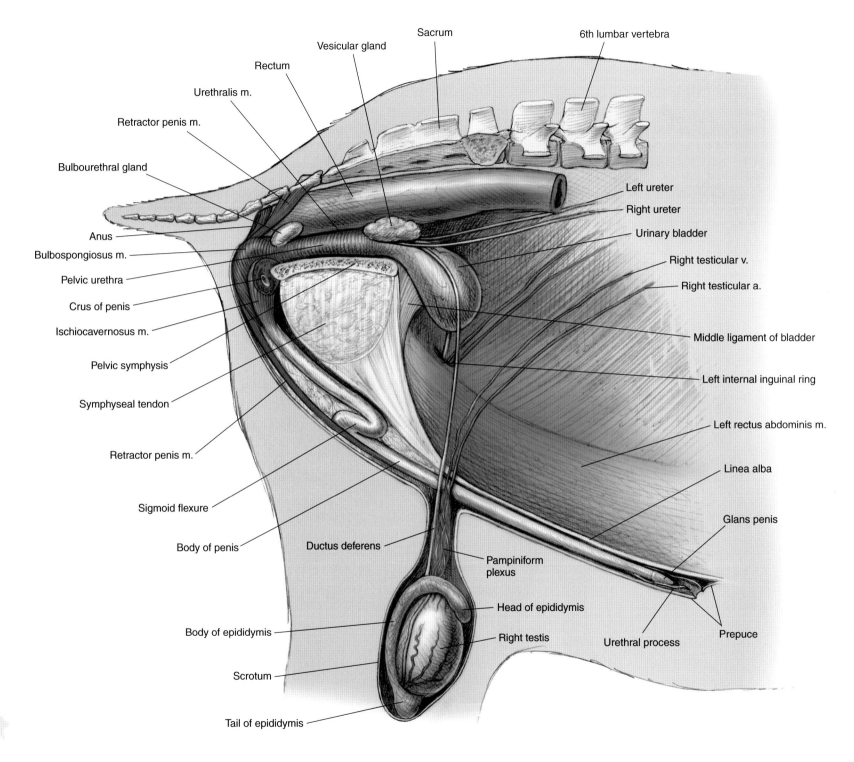

Sacrum

6th lumbar vertebra

Vesicular gland

Rectum

Urethralis m.

Retractor penis m.

Bulbourethral gland

Left ureter

Right ureter

Anus

Urinary bladder

Bulbospongiosus m.

Right testicular v.

Pelvic urethra

Right testicular a.

Crus of penis

Ischiocavernosus m.

Middle ligament of bladder

Pelvic symphysis

Left internal inguinal ring

Symphyseal tendon

Left rectus abdominis m.

Retractor penis m.

Linea alba

Sigmoid flexure

Body of penis

Ductus deferens

Glans penis

Pampiniform
plexus

Head of epididymis

Prepuce

Body of epididymis

Right testis

Urethral process

Scrotum

Tail of epididymis

**PLATE 4.15**    Relations of the reproductive organs of the buck. Right pelvic limb and
body wall are removed. Right lateral view. a = artery, m = muscle, v = vein

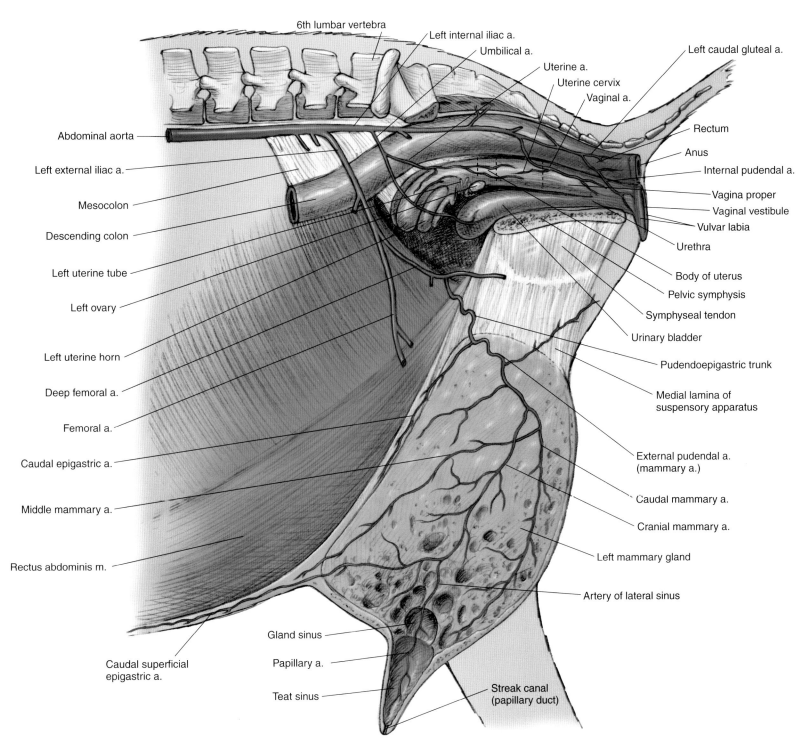

6th lumbar vertebra

Left internal iliac a.

Umbilical a.

Uterine a.

Uterine cervix

Vaginal a.

Left caudal gluteal a.

Abdominal aorta

Left external iliac a.

Mesocolon

Descending colon

Left uterine tube

Left ovary

Left uterine horn

Deep femoral a.

Femoral a.

Caudal epigastric a.

Middle mammary a.

Rectus abdominis m.

Caudal superficial
epigastric a.

Rectum

Anus

Internal pudendal a.

Vagina proper

Vaginal vestibule

Vulvar labia

Urethra

Body of uterus

Pelvic symphysis

Symphyseal tendon

Urinary bladder

Pudendoepigastric trunk

Medial lamina of
suspensory apparatus

External pudendal a.
(mammary a.)

Caudal mammary a.

Cranial mammary a.

Left mammary gland

Artery of lateral sinus

Gland sinus

Papillary a.

Teat sinus

Streak canal
(papillary duct)

**87**

**PLATE 4.16** Relations of the reproductive organs of the doe.
Median section. a = artery, m = muscle

# SECTION 5   THE LLAMA AND ALPACA
## (*Lama glama* and *Lama pacos*)

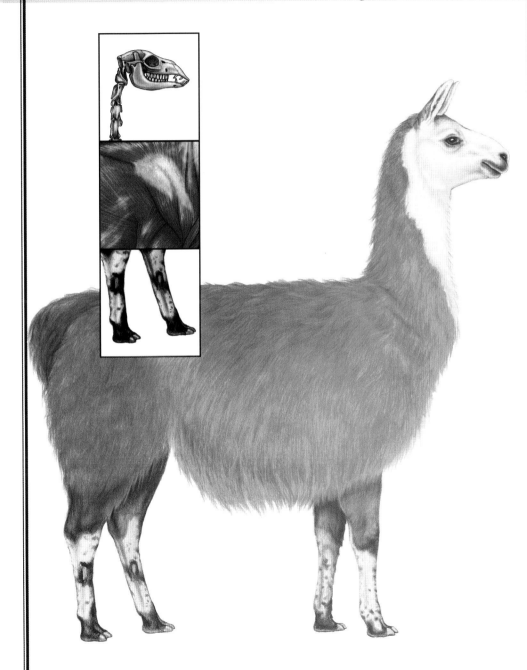

## PLATES

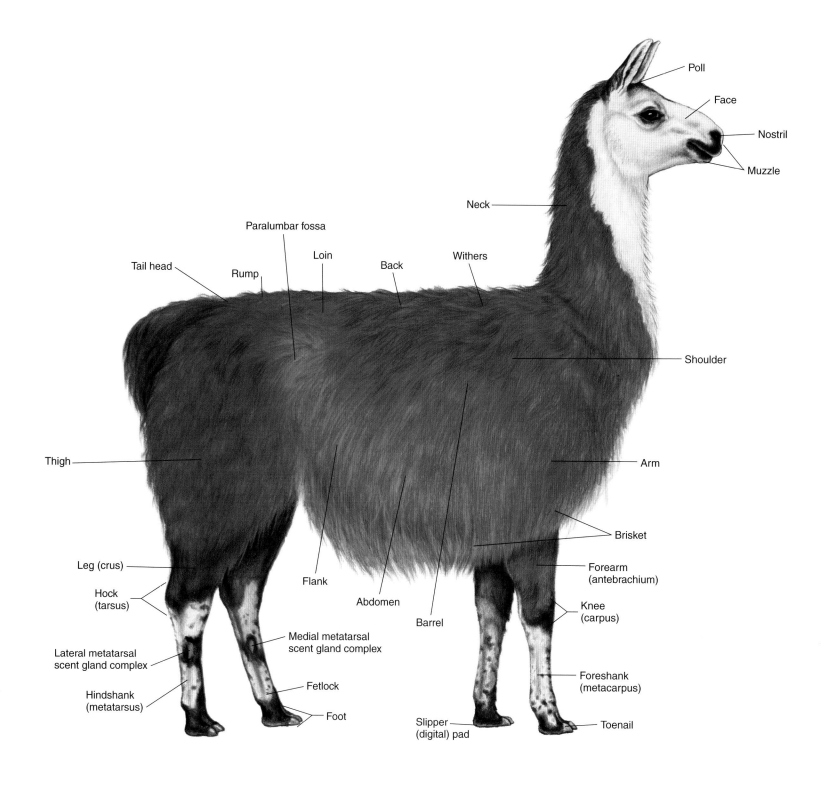

Poll

Face

Nostril

Muzzle

Neck

Paralumbar fossa

Loin

Back

Withers

Tail head

Rump

Shoulder

Thigh

Arm

Brisket

Leg (crus)

Forearm
(antebrachium)

Hock
(tarsus)

Flank

Abdomen

Barrel

Knee
(carpus)

Lateral metatarsal
scent gland complex

Medial metatarsal
scent gland complex

Hindshank
(metatarsus)

Fetlock

Foreshank
(metacarpus)

Foot

Slipper
(digital) pad

Toenail

90

**PLATE 5.1**  Right lateral view of a male llama.

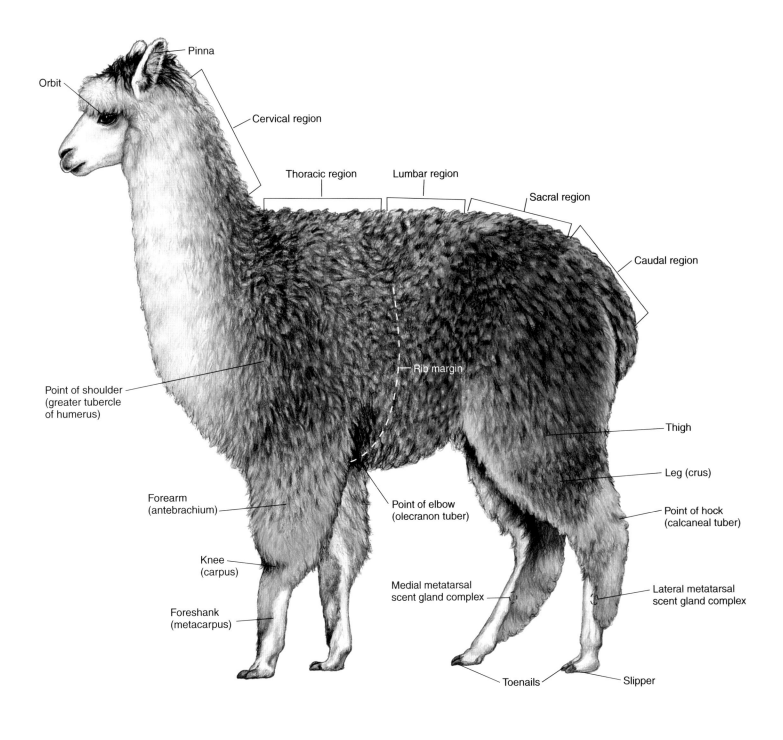

Pinna

Orbit

Cervical region

Thoracic region

Lumbar region

Sacral region

Caudal region

Rib margin

Point of shoulder
(greater tubercle
of humerus)

Thigh

Leg (crus)

Forearm
(antebrachium)

Point of elbow
(olecranon tuber)

Point of hock
(calcaneal tuber)

Knee
(carpus)

Medial metatarsal
scent gland complex

Lateral metatarsal
scent gland complex

Foreshank
(metacarpus)

Toenails

Slipper

**PLATE 5.2** Left lateral view of a female huacaya alpaca. Dorsal vertebral regions are indicated.

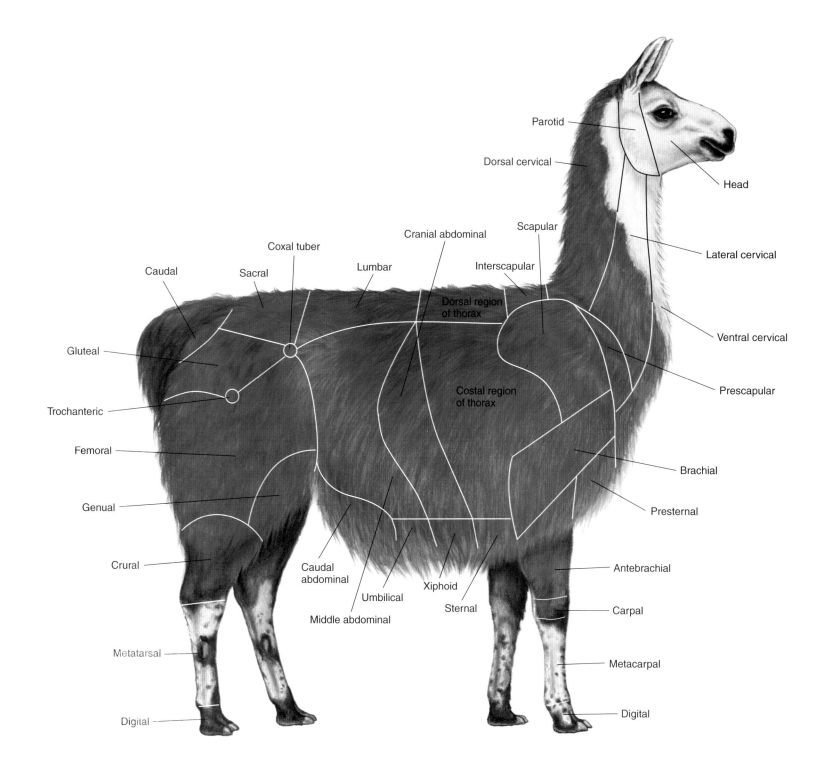

**PLATE 5.3** Body regions of the llama.

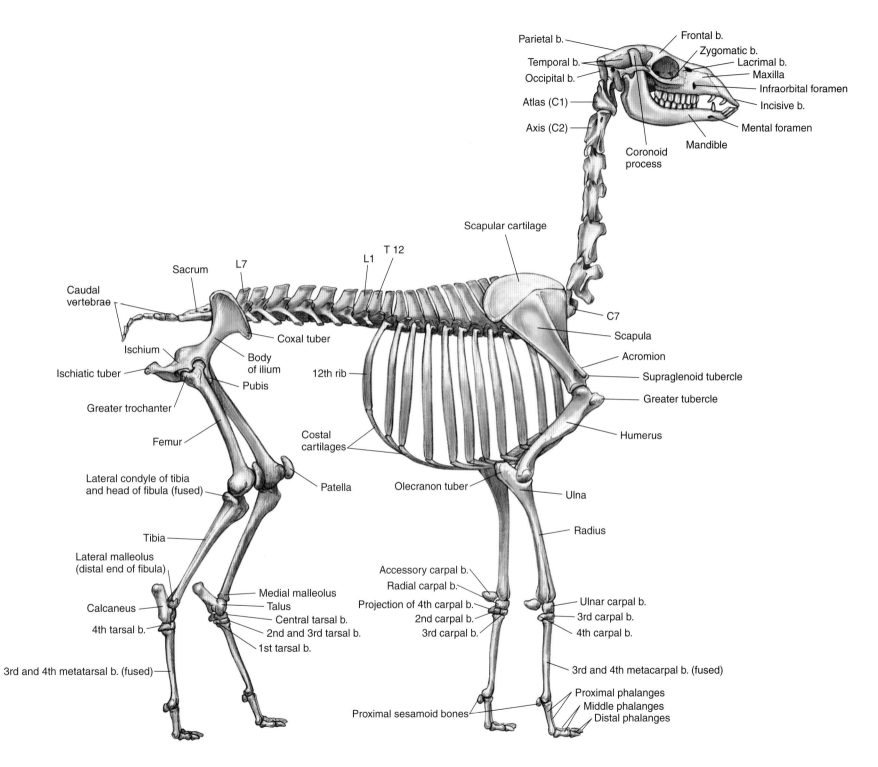

**PLATE 5.4**  Skeleton of the llama.  Right lateral view.  C = cervical vertebra,
T = thoracic vertebra, L = lumbar vetebra,  b = bone

93

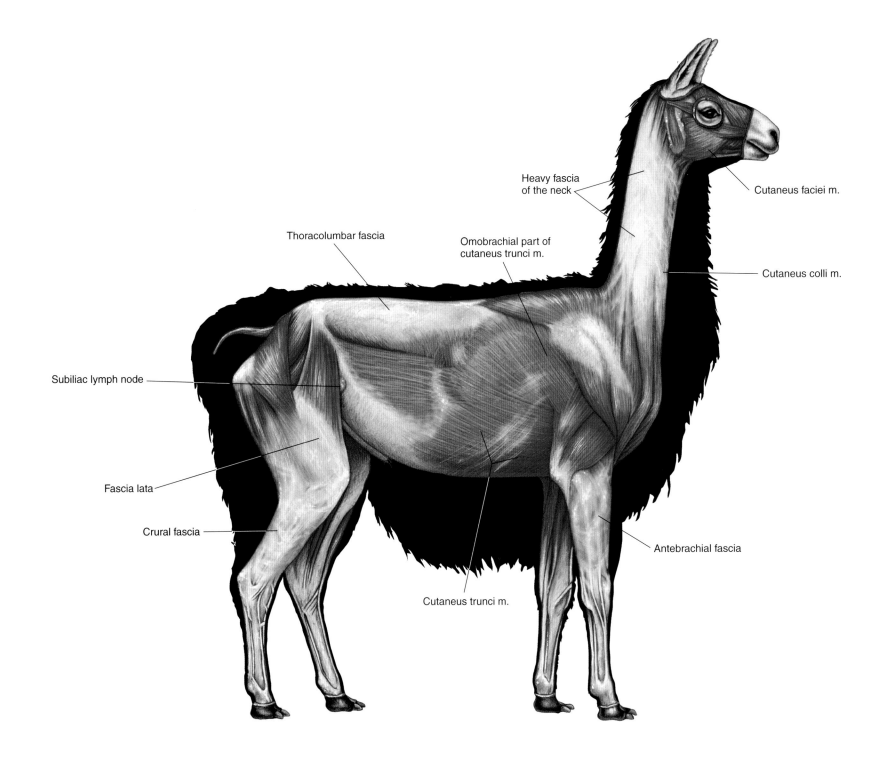

Heavy fascia
of the neck

Cutaneus faciei m.

Thoracolumbar fascia

Omobrachial part of
cutaneus trunci m.

Cutaneus colli m.

Subiliac lymph node

Fascia lata

Crural fascia

Antebrachial fascia

Cutaneus trunci m.

94

**PLATE** 5.5   Cutaneous muscles and major fasciae of the male llama.
Right lateral view. m = muscle

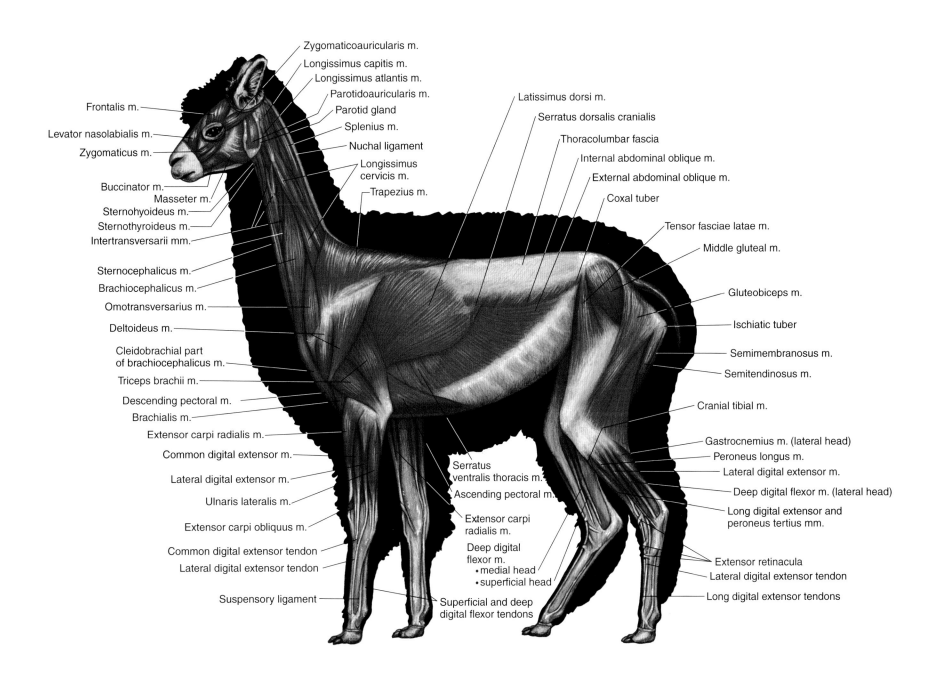

Zygomaticoauricularis m.
Longissimus capitis m.
Longissimus atlantis m.
Parotidoauricularis m.
Parotid gland
Splenius m.
Nuchal ligament
Longissimus cervicis m.
Trapezius m.

Frontalis m.
Levator nasolabialis m.
Zygomaticus m.
Buccinator m.
Masseter m.
Sternohyoideus m.
Sternothyroideus m.
Intertransversarii mm.
Sternocephalicus m.
Brachiocephalicus m.
Omotransversarius m.
Deltoideus m.
Cleidobrachial part of brachiocephalicus m.
Triceps brachii m.
Descending pectoral m.
Brachialis m.
Extensor carpi radialis m.
Common digital extensor m.
Lateral digital extensor m.
Ulnaris lateralis m.
Extensor carpi obliquus m.
Common digital extensor tendon
Lateral digital extensor tendon
Suspensory ligament

Latissimus dorsi m.
Serratus dorsalis cranialis
Thoracolumbar fascia
Internal abdominal oblique m.
External abdominal oblique m.
Coxal tuber
Tensor fasciae latae m.
Middle gluteal m.
Gluteobiceps m.
Ischiatic tuber
Semimembranosus m.
Semitendinosus m.
Cranial tibial m.
Gastrocnemius m. (lateral head)
Peroneus longus m.
Lateral digital extensor m.
Deep digital flexor m. (lateral head)
Long digital extensor and peroneus tertius mm.
Extensor retinacula
Lateral digital extensor tendon
Long digital extensor tendons

Serratus ventralis thoracis m.
Ascending pectoral m.
Extensor carpi radialis m.
Deep digital flexor m.
• medial head
• superficial head
Superficial and deep digital flexor tendons

95

**PLATE 5.6**  Superficial muscles of the female alpaca.  Left lateral view. m = muscle

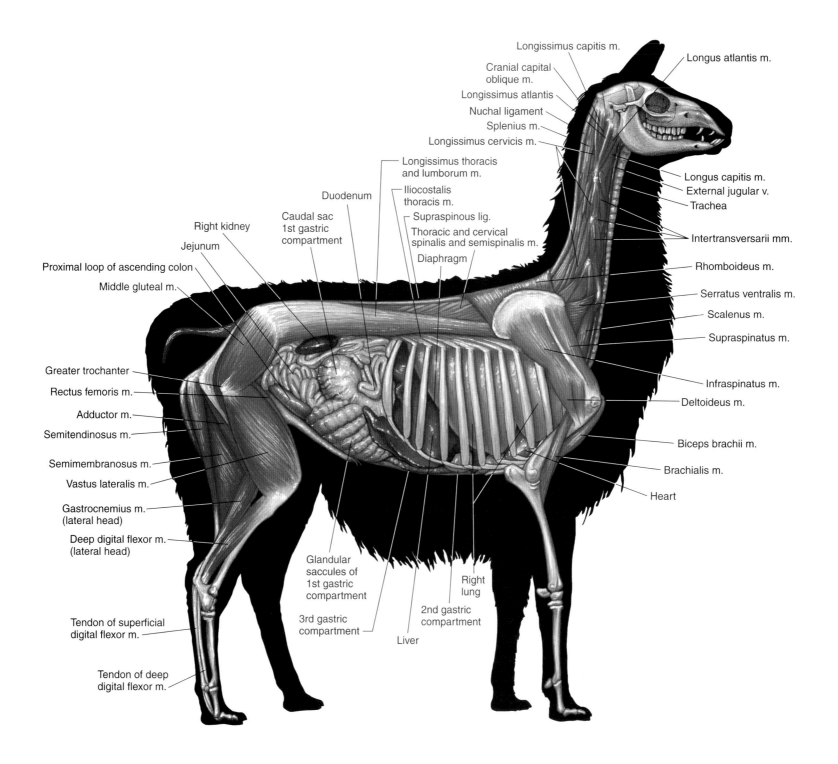

Longissimus capitis m.

Longus atlantis m.

Cranial capital
oblique m.

Longissimus atlantis

Nuchal ligament

Splenius m.

Longissimus cervicis m.

Longissimus thoracis
and lumborum m.

Duodenum

Iliocostalis
thoracis m.

Caudal sac
1st gastric
compartment

Supraspinous lig.

Right kidney

Thoracic and cervical
spinalis and semispinalis m.

Jejunum

Diaphragm

Proximal loop of ascending colon

Middle gluteal m.

Longus capitis m.

External jugular v.

Trachea

Intertransversarii mm.

Rhomboideus m.

Serratus ventralis m.

Scalenus m.

Supraspinatus m.

Greater trochanter

Rectus femoris m.

Adductor m.

Semitendinosus m.

Infraspinatus m.

Deltoideus m.

Semimembranosus m.

Vastus lateralis m.

Biceps brachii m.

Brachialis m.

Gastrocnemius m.
(lateral head)

Deep digital flexor m.
(lateral head)

Heart

Glandular
saccules of
1st gastric
compartment

Right
lung

Tendon of superficial
digital flexor m.

3rd gastric
compartment

2nd gastric
compartment

Liver

Tendon of deep
digital flexor m.

**PLATE 5.7** Deep muscles and *in situ* viscera of the male llama. Omentum is removed.
Right lateral view. m = muscle, v = vein, lig = ligament

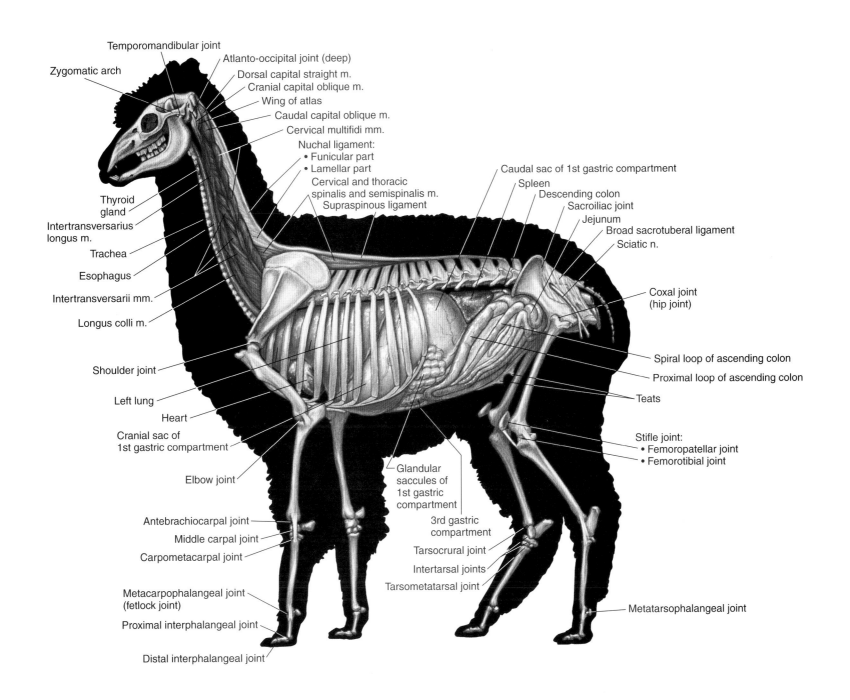

Temporomandibular joint

Atlanto-occipital joint (deep)

Zygomatic arch

Dorsal capital straight m.

Cranial capital oblique m.

Wing of atlas

Caudal capital oblique m.

Cervical multifidi mm.

Nuchal ligament:
• Funicular part
• Lamellar part

Cervical and thoracic
spinalis and semispinalis m.

Supraspinous ligament

Thyroid
gland

Intertransversarius
longus m.

Trachea

Esophagus

Intertransversarii mm.

Longus colli m.

Shoulder joint

Left lung

Heart

Cranial sac of
1st gastric compartment

Elbow joint

Antebrachiocarpal joint

Middle carpal joint

Carpometacarpal joint

Metacarpophalangeal joint
(fetlock joint)

Proximal interphalangeal joint

Distal interphalangeal joint

Glandular
saccules of
1st gastric
compartment

3rd gastric
compartment

Tarsocrural joint

Intertarsal joints

Tarsometatarsal joint

Caudal sac of 1st gastric compartment

Spleen

Descending colon

Sacroiliac joint

Jejunum

Broad sacrotuberal ligament

Sciatic n.

Coxal joint
(hip joint)

Spiral loop of ascending colon

Proximal loop of ascending colon

Teats

Stifle joint:
• Femoropatellar joint
• Femorotibial joint

Metatarsophalangeal joint

97

**PLATE 5.8**   Deep cervical muscles, *in situ* viscera, and major joints of the female alpaca.
The omentum is removed.  Left lateral view. m = muscle

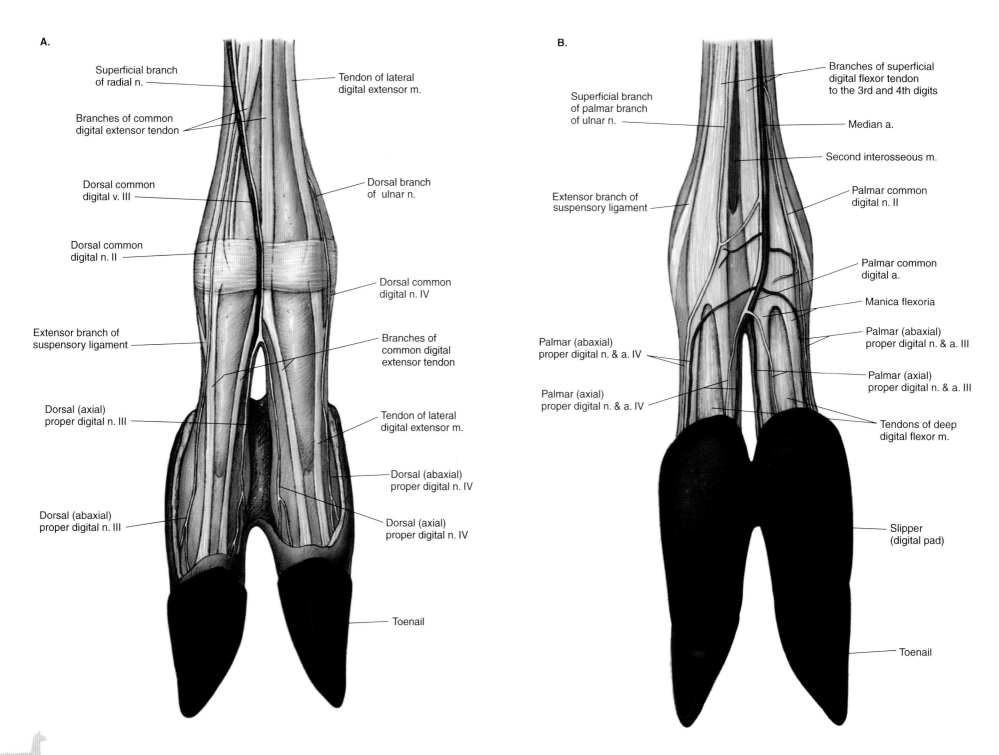

**A.**

Superficial branch
of radial n.

Branches of common
digital extensor tendon

Dorsal common
digital v. III

Dorsal common
digital n. II

Extensor branch of
suspensory ligament

Dorsal (axial)
proper digital n. III

Dorsal (abaxial)
proper digital n. III

Tendon of lateral
digital extensor m.

Dorsal branch
of ulnar n.

Dorsal common
digital n. IV

Branches of
common digital
extensor tendon

Tendon of lateral
digital extensor m.

Dorsal (abaxial)
proper digital n. IV

Dorsal (axial)
proper digital n. IV

Toenail

**B.**

Superficial branch
of palmar branch
of ulnar n.

Extensor branch of
suspensory ligament

Palmar (abaxial)
proper digital n. & a. IV

Palmar (axial)
proper digital n. & a. IV

Branches of superficial
digital flexor tendon
to the 3rd and 4th digits

Median a.

Second interosseous m.

Palmar common
digital n. II

Palmar common
digital a.

Manica flexoria

Palmar (abaxial)
proper digital n. & a. III

Palmar (axial)
proper digital n. & a. III

Tendons of deep
digital flexor m.

Slipper
(digital pad)

Toenail

**PLATE 5.9**  Major structures of the lamoid left distal metacarpus and digits.  **A.** Dorsal view.
**B.** Palmar view. n = nerve, v = vein, m = muscle, a = artery

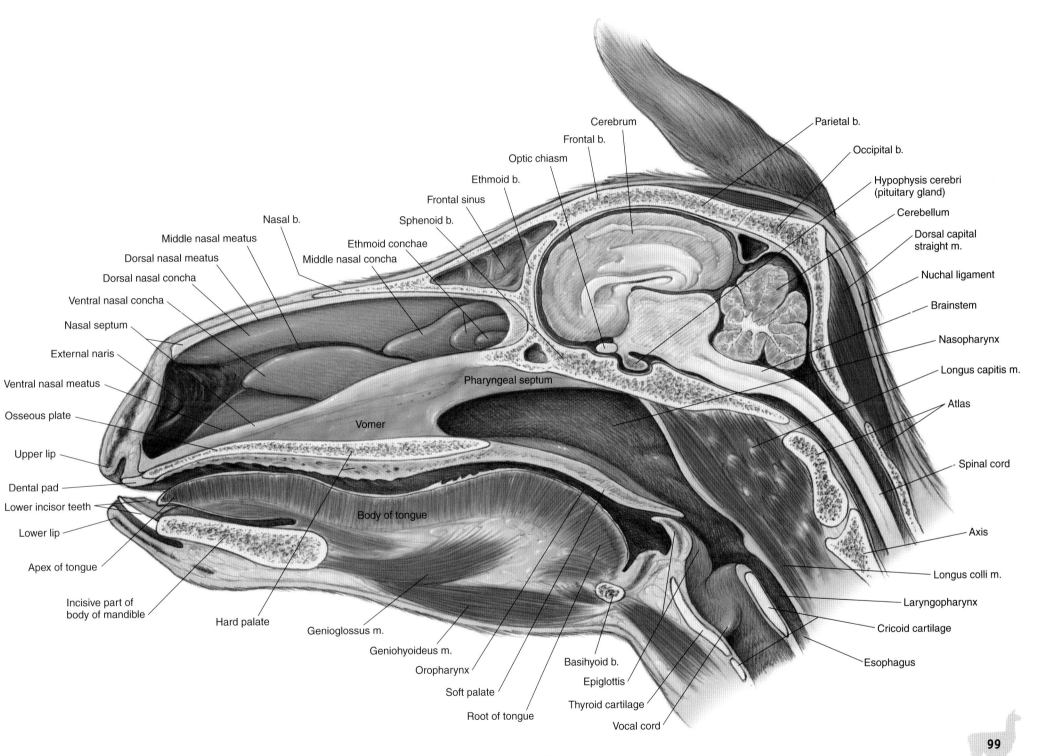

**PLATE 5.10**  Median section of the llama's head. Most of the nasal septum is removed. b = bone, m = muscle

Cerebrum

Frontal b.

Optic chiasm

Ethmoid b.

Frontal sinus

Sphenoid b.

Ethmoid conchae

Middle nasal concha

Nasal b.

Middle nasal meatus

Dorsal nasal meatus

Dorsal nasal concha

Ventral nasal concha

Nasal septum

External naris

Ventral nasal meatus

Osseous plate

Upper lip

Dental pad

Lower incisor teeth

Lower lip

Apex of tongue

Incisive part of
body of mandible

Hard palate

Genioglossus m.

Geniohyoideus m.

Oropharynx

Soft palate

Root of tongue

Basihyoid b.

Epiglottis

Thyroid cartilage

Vocal cord

Body of tongue

Vomer

Pharyngeal septum

Parietal b.

Occipital b.

Hypophysis cerebri
(pituitary gland)

Cerebellum

Dorsal capital
straight m.

Nuchal ligament

Brainstem

Nasopharynx

Longus capitis m.

Atlas

Spinal cord

Axis

Longus colli m.

Laryngopharynx

Cricoid cartilage

Esophagus

**99**

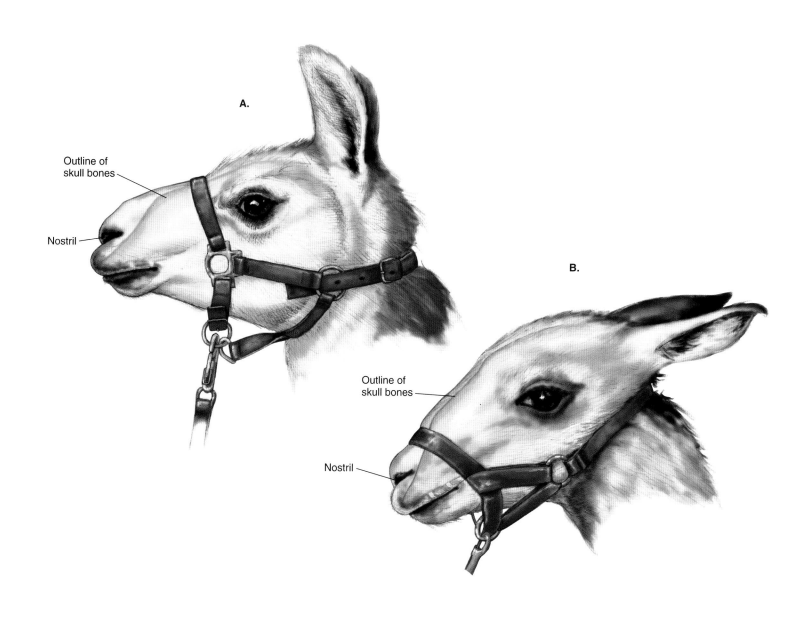

A.

Outline of
skull bones

Nostril

B.

Outline of
skull bones

Nostril

**PLATE 5.11** **A**. Proper placement of a halter on a llama's head. **B.** Improper placement
of a halter. Pressure on the nostrils interferes with breathing.

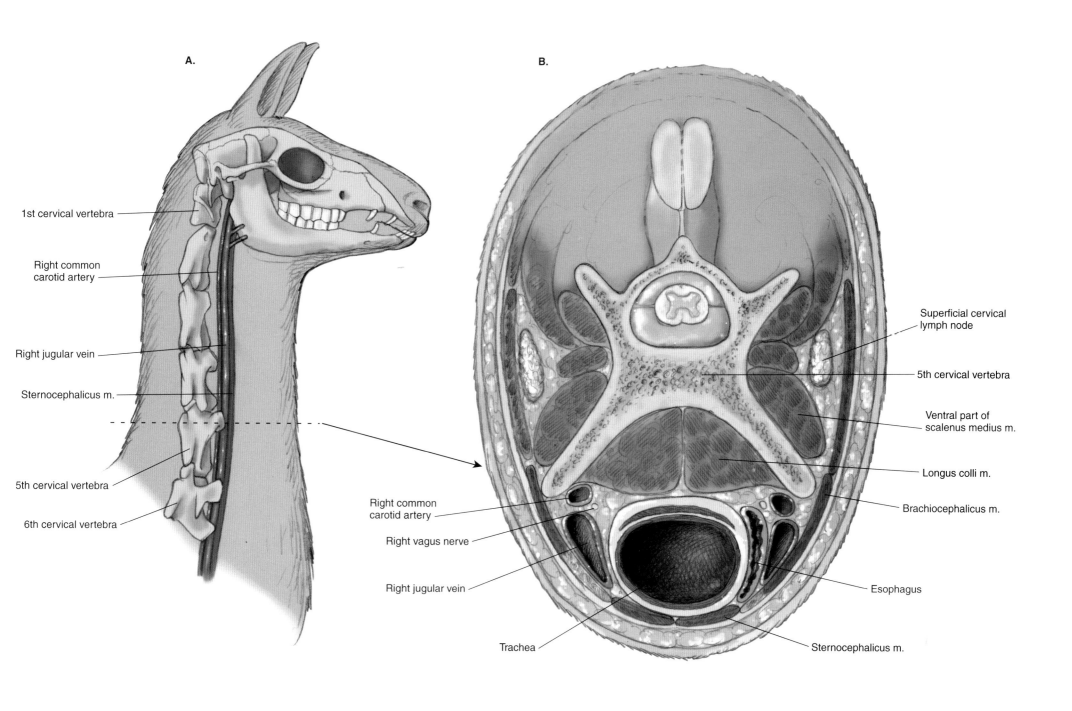

A.

1st cervical vertebra

Right common
carotid artery

Right jugular vein

Sternocephalicus m.

5th cervical vertebra

6th cervical vertebra

B.

Superficial cervical
lymph node

5th cervical vertebra

Ventral part of
scalenus medius m.

Longus colli m.

Brachiocephalicus m.

Right common
carotid artery

Right vagus nerve

Right jugular vein

Trachea

Esophagus

Sternocephalicus m.

**PLATE 5.12** Relations of the llama's common carotid artery and jugular vein. **A.** Right lateral view of the head and neck. **B.** Cross-section through the neck at the level of the 5th cervical vertebra. m = muscle

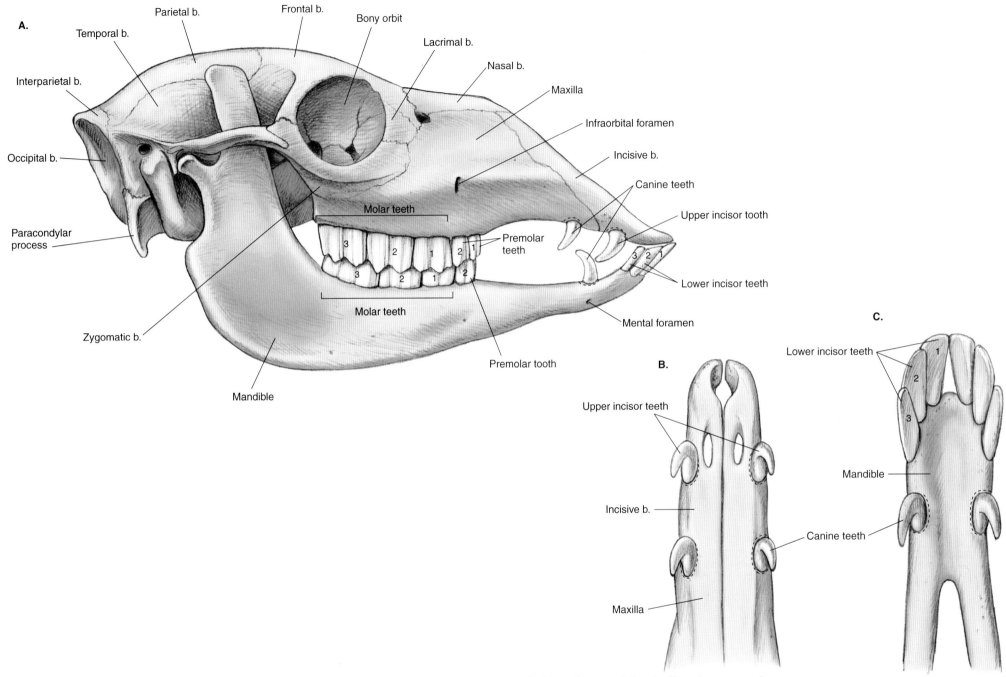

**PLATE 5.13** Dentition of the male llama. **A.** Right lateral view of the skull and crowns of permanent teeth *in situ*. **B.** Ventral view of the crowns of the upper incisor and canine teeth. **C.** Dorsal view of the crowns of the lower incisor and canine teeth. *Dashed lines* indicate the plane of sectioning (2–3 mm above the gum [gingival] line) for cutting off the crowns of deciduous or erupting permanent canine and upper incisor teeth. b = bone

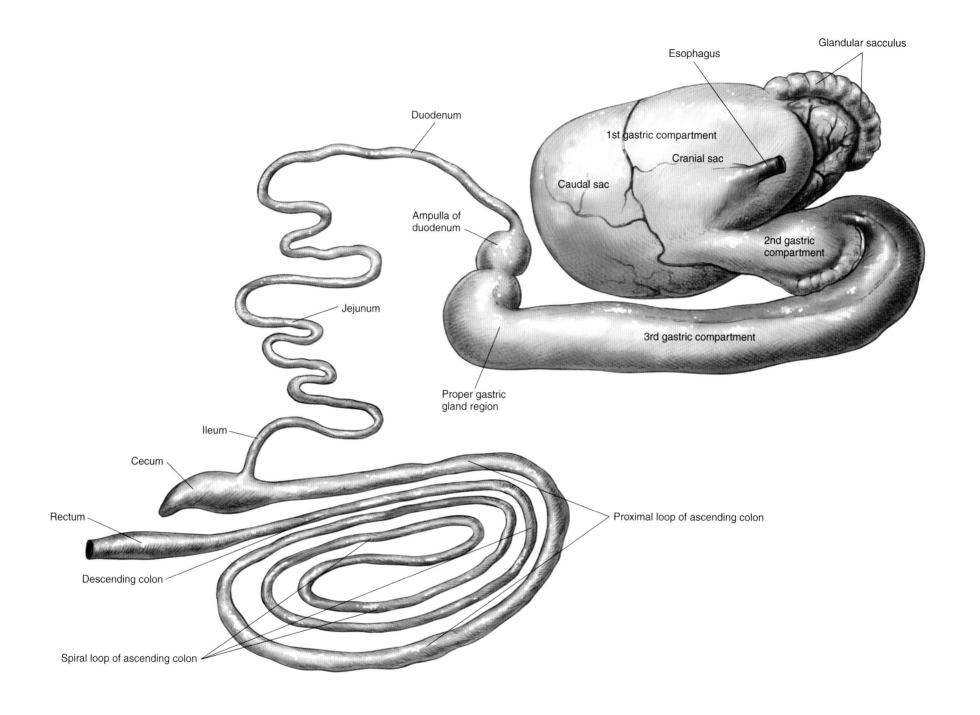

Esophagus

Glandular sacculus

Duodenum

1st gastric compartment

Cranial sac

Caudal sac

2nd gastric compartment

Ampulla of duodenum

3rd gastric compartment

Jejunum

Proper gastric gland region

Ileum

Cecum

Proximal loop of ascending colon

Rectum

Descending colon

Spiral loop of ascending colon

**103**

**PLATE 5.14** Isolated stomach and intestines of the male llama. Jejunum is shortened.

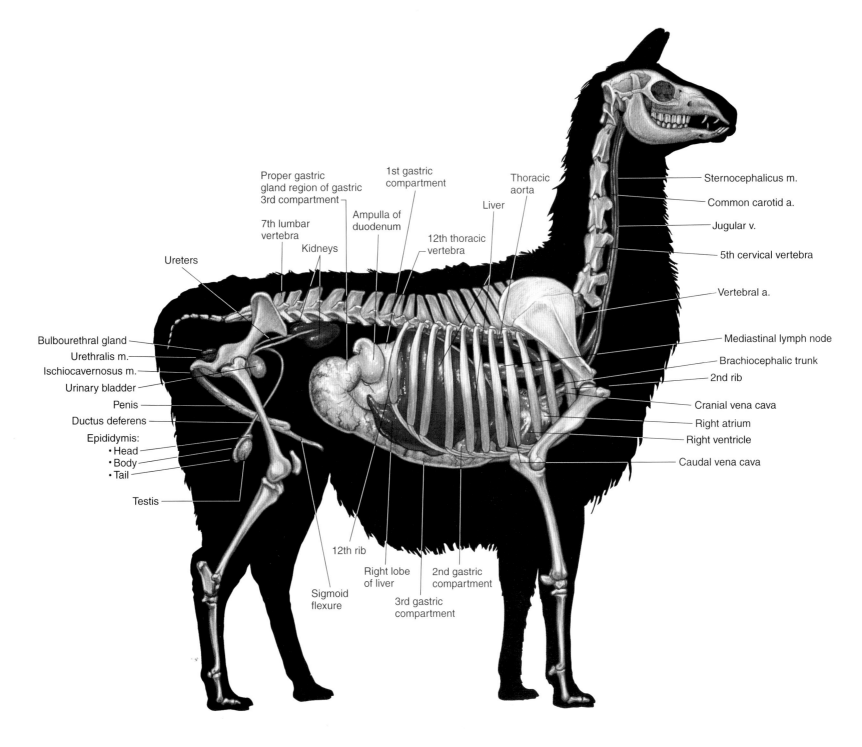

Proper gastric gland region of gastric 3rd compartment

7th lumbar vertebra

Kidneys

Ureters

1st gastric compartment

Ampulla of duodenum

12th thoracic vertebra

Thoracic aorta

Liver

Sternocephalicus m.

Common carotid a.

Jugular v.

5th cervical vertebra

Vertebral a.

Mediastinal lymph node

Brachiocephalic trunk

2nd rib

Cranial vena cava

Right atrium

Right ventricle

Caudal vena cava

Bulbourethral gland

Urethralis m.

Ischiocavernosus m.

Urinary bladder

Penis

Ductus deferens

Epididymis:
• Head
• Body
• Tail

Testis

12th rib

Sigmoid flexure

Right lobe of liver

2nd gastric compartment

3rd gastric compartment

**PLATE 5.15** Reproductive and urinary organs, stomach, liver, heart, and adjacent major vessels related to the skeleton of the male llama. Lungs and intestines are removed. Right lateral view. v = vein, a = artery, m = muscle

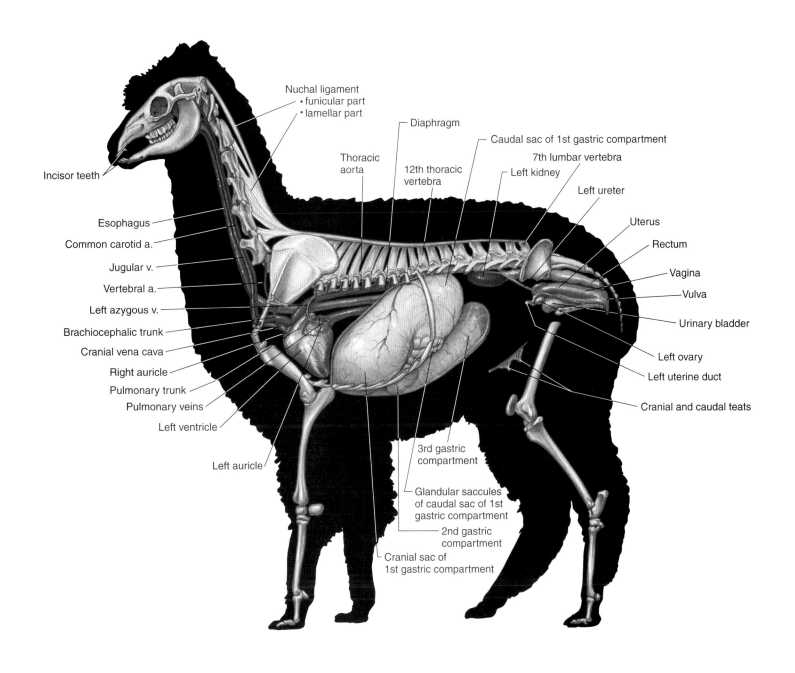

Nuchal ligament
• funicular part
• lamellar part

Diaphragm

Caudal sac of 1st gastric compartment

Thoracic aorta

12th thoracic vertebra

7th lumbar vertebra

Left kidney

Left ureter

Uterus

Rectum

Vagina

Vulva

Urinary bladder

Left ovary

Left uterine duct

Cranial and caudal teats

Incisor teeth

Esophagus

Common carotid a.

Jugular v.

Vertebral a.

Left azygous v.

Brachiocephalic trunk

Cranial vena cava

Right auricle

Pulmonary trunk

Pulmonary veins

Left ventricle

Left auricle

3rd gastric compartment

Glandular saccules of caudal sac of 1st gastric compartment

2nd gastric compartment

Cranial sac of 1st gastric compartment

**PLATE 5.16**    Reproductive and urinary organs, stomach, heart, and adjacent major vessels of the female alpaca. Lungs and intestines are removed.  Left lateral view. a = artery, v = vein

105

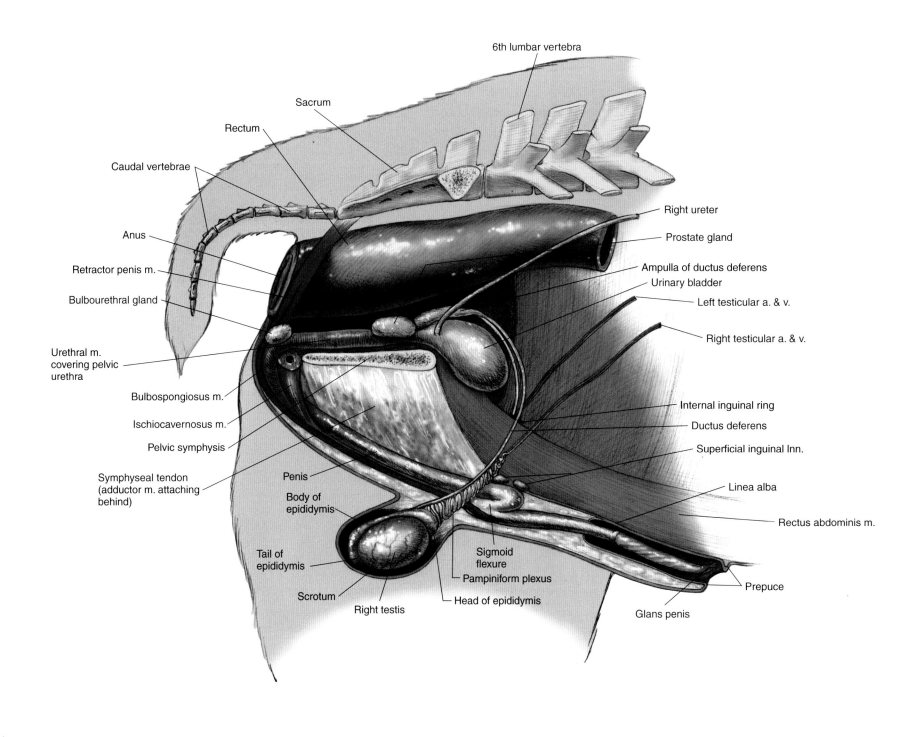

6th lumbar vertebra

Sacrum

Rectum

Caudal vertebrae

Anus

Retractor penis m.

Bulbourethral gland

Urethral m.
covering pelvic
urethra

Bulbospongiosus m.

Ischiocavernosus m.

Pelvic symphysis

Symphyseal tendon
(adductor m. attaching
behind)

Penis

Body of
epididymis

Tail of
epididymis

Scrotum

Right testis

Sigmoid
flexure

Pampiniform plexus

Head of epididymis

Right ureter

Prostate gland

Ampulla of ductus deferens

Urinary bladder

Left testicular a. & v.

Right testicular a. & v.

Internal inguinal ring

Ductus deferens

Superficial inguinal lnn.

Linea alba

Rectus abdominis m.

Prepuce

Glans penis

**PLATE 5.17** Relations of the reproductive organs of the male llama. Right lateral view.
m = muscle, lnn = lymph nodes, v = vein, a = artery

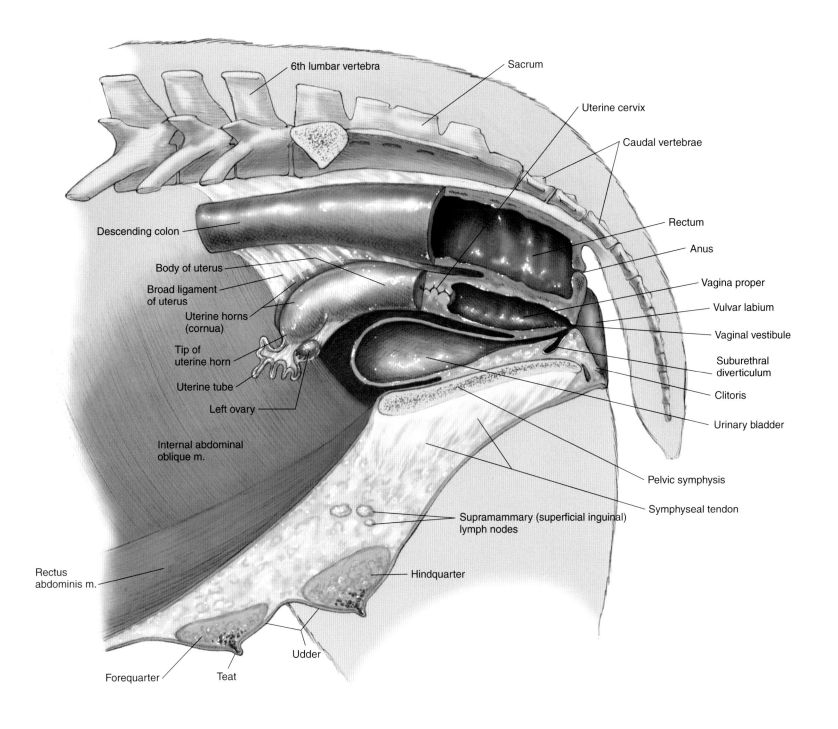

6th lumbar vertebra

Sacrum

Uterine cervix

Caudal vertebrae

Descending colon

Rectum

Anus

Body of uterus

Vagina proper

Broad ligament of uterus

Vulvar labium

Uterine horns (cornua)

Vaginal vestibule

Tip of uterine horn

Suburethral diverticulum

Uterine tube

Clitoris

Left ovary

Urinary bladder

Internal abdominal oblique m.

Pelvic symphysis

Symphyseal tendon

Supramammary (superficial inguinal) lymph nodes

Rectus abdominis m.

Hindquarter

Forequarter

Teat

Udder

**PLATE 5.18**   Relations of the reproductive organs of the female alpaca.
Partial median section.  Left lateral view. m = muscle

# SECTION 6 THE SWINE *(Sus scrofa domesticus)*

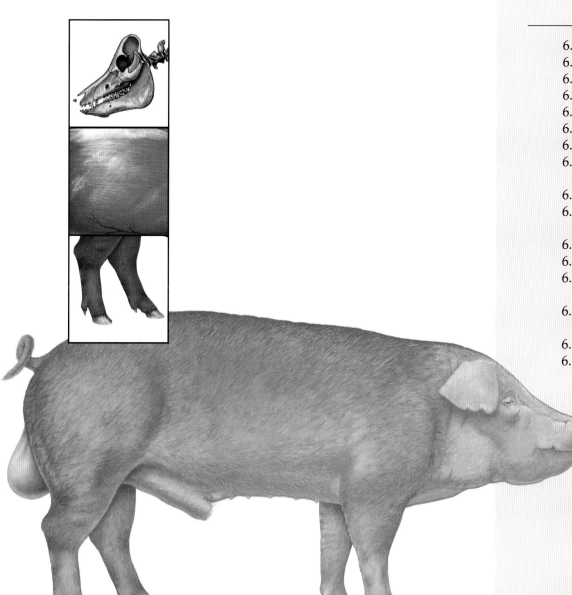

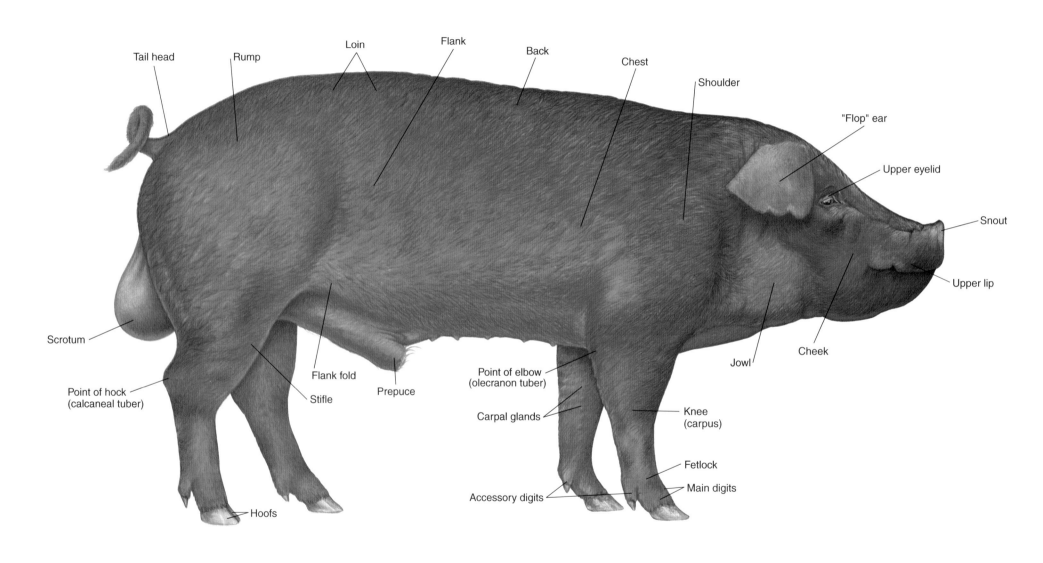

**PLATE 6.1** Right lateral view of a boar.

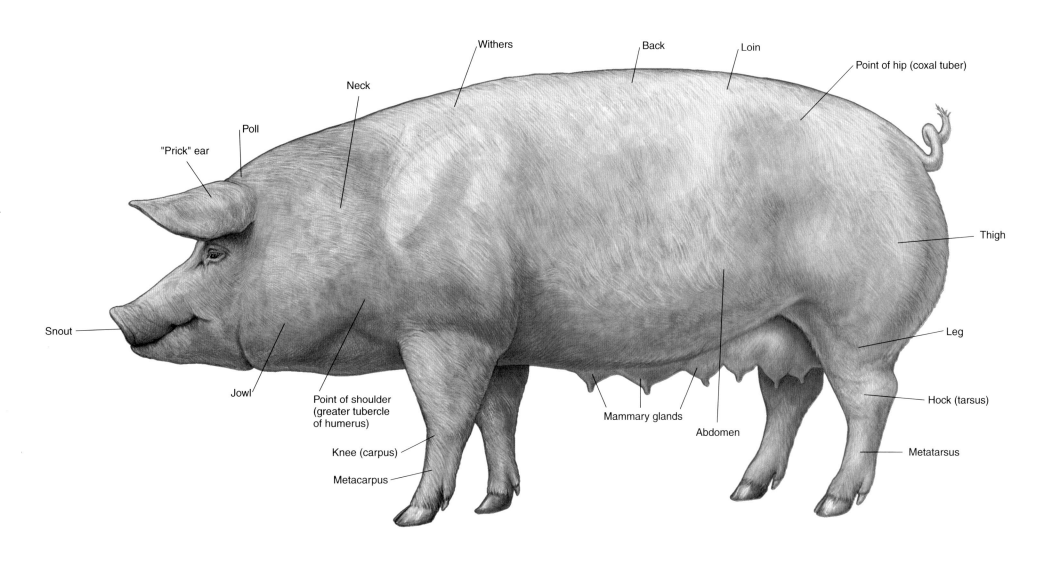

**PLATE 6.2** Left lateral view of a sow.

**111**

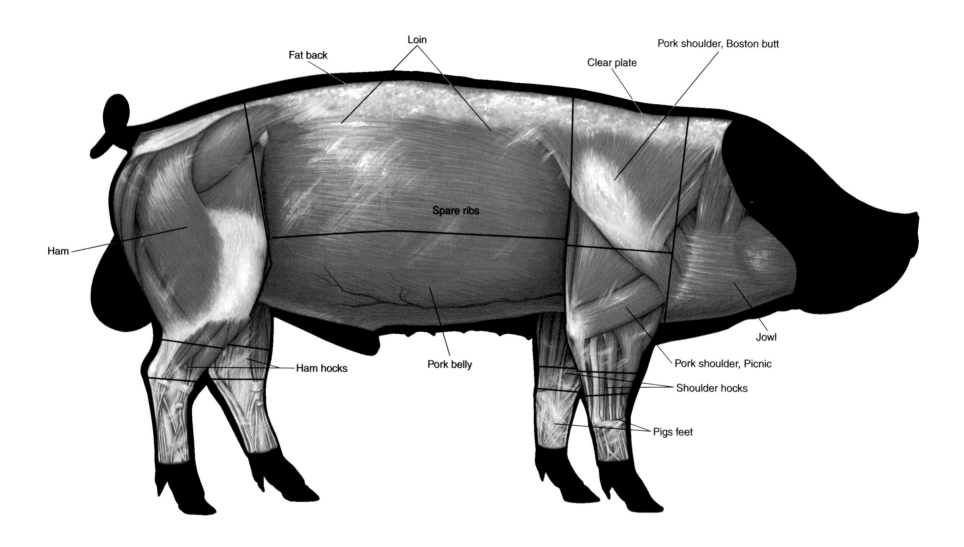

Loin

Fat back

Pork shoulder, Boston butt

Clear plate

Spare ribs

Ham

Jowl

Ham hocks

Pork belly

Pork shoulder, Picnic

Shoulder hocks

Pigs feet

**PLATE 6.3** Carcass cuts of the hog.

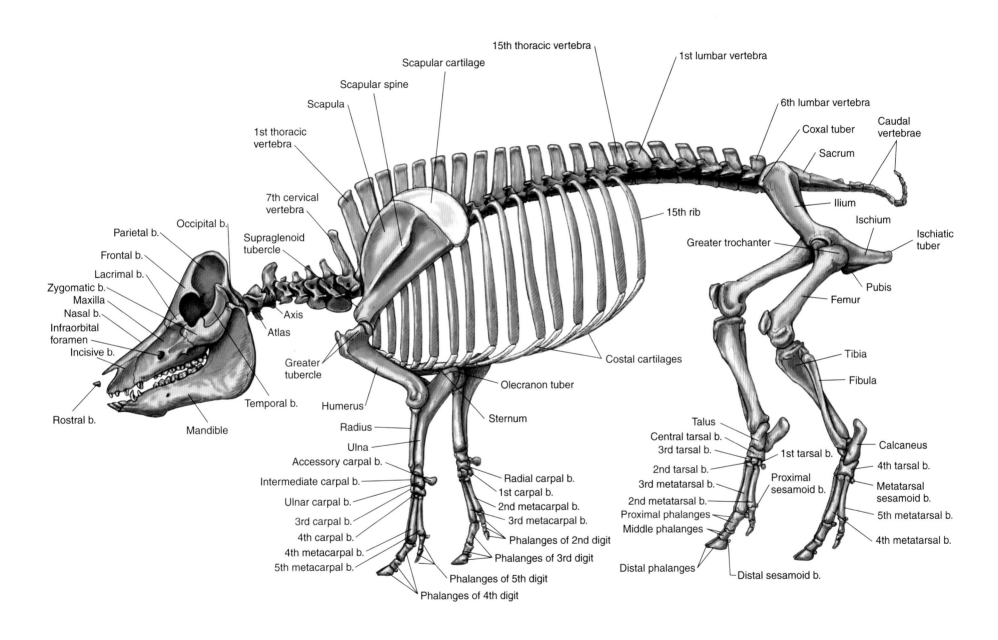

**PLATE 6.4**  Skeleton of the swine. b = bone

113

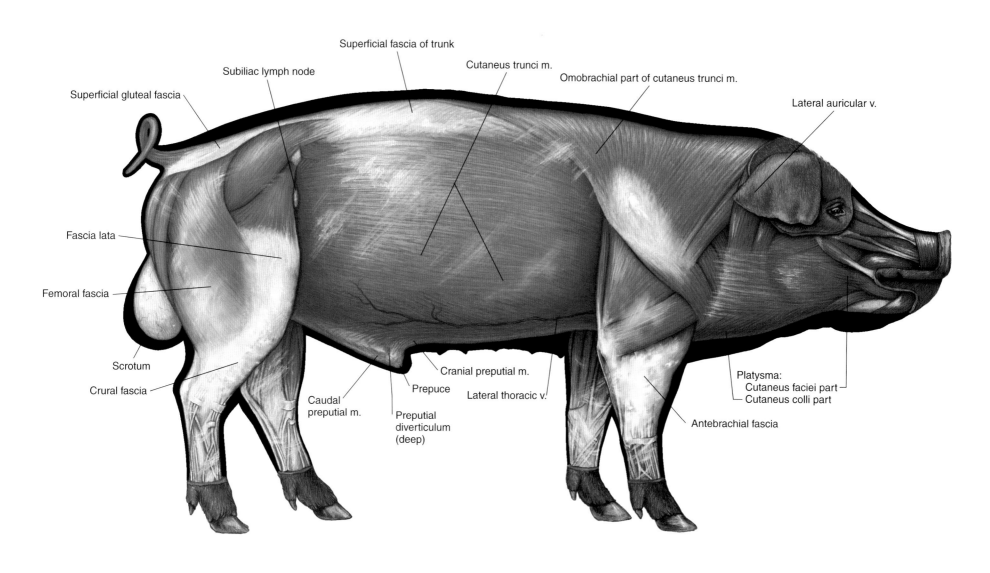

Superficial fascia of trunk

Subiliac lymph node

Cutaneus trunci m.

Omobrachial part of cutaneus trunci m.

Superficial gluteal fascia

Lateral auricular v.

Fascia lata

Femoral fascia

Scrotum

Crural fascia

Caudal preputial m.

Preputial diverticulum (deep)

Prepuce

Cranial preputial m.

Lateral thoracic v.

Platysma:
Cutaneus faciei part
Cutaneus colli part

Antebrachial fascia

**PLATE 6.5**   Cutaneous and superficial muscles of the boar. Panniculus adiposus (fat layer) removed.  Right lateral view. v = vein, m = muscle

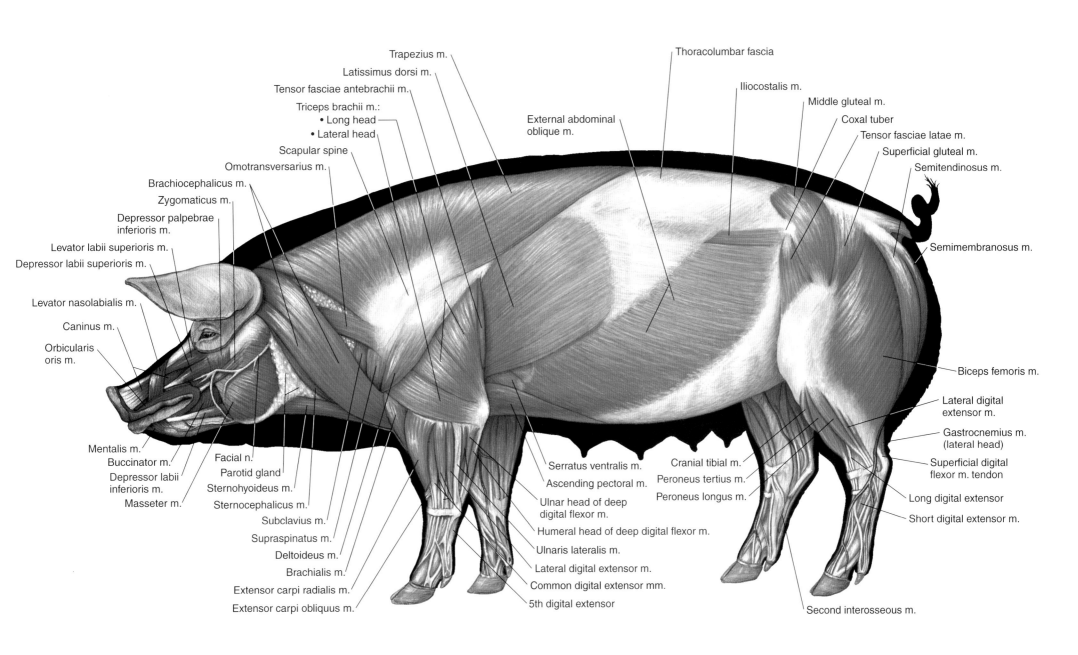

**PLATE 6.6** Superficial muscles of the sow. Left lateral view. m = muscle, n = nerve

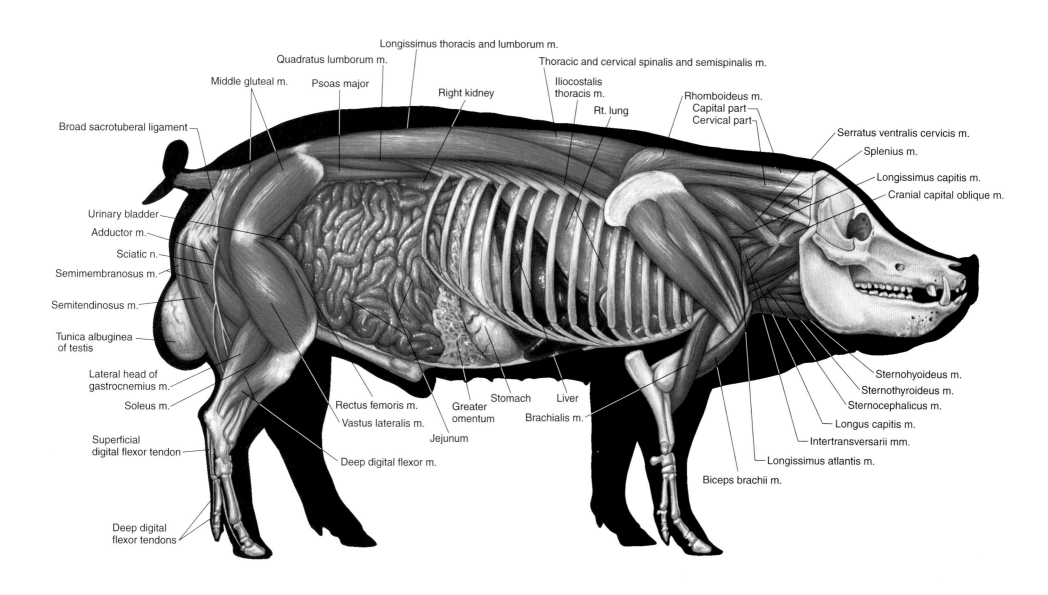

**PLATE 6.7**  Deep muscles and *in situ* viscera of the boar.
Right lateral view. m = muscle, n = nerve

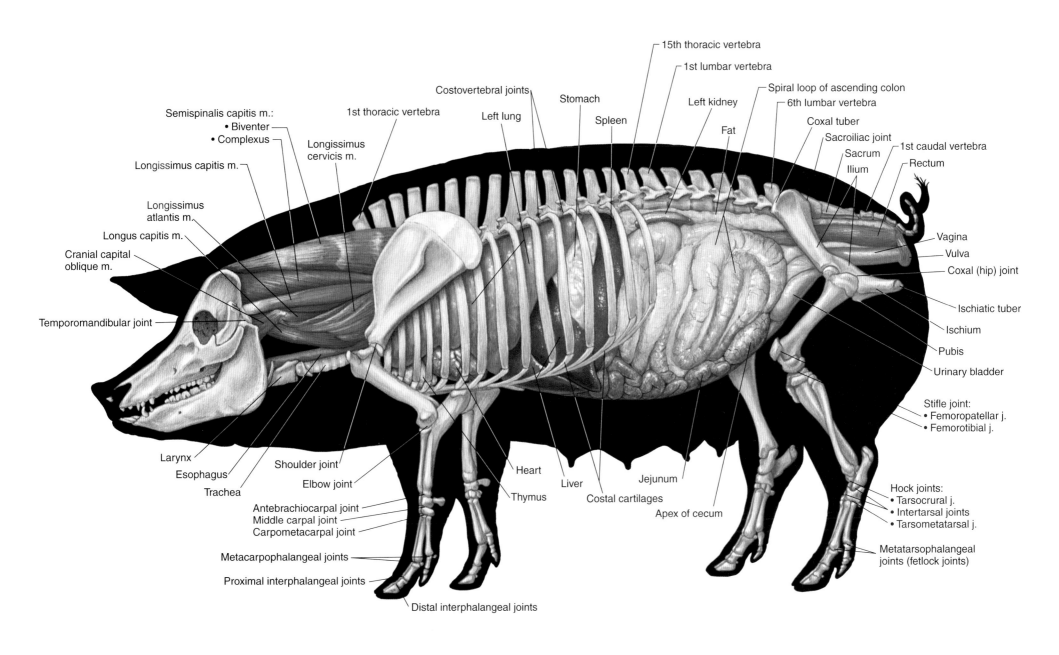

Semispinalis capitis m.:
• Biventer
• Complexus

Longissimus capitis m.

Longissimus atlantis m.

Longus capitis m.

Cranial capital oblique m.

Temporomandibular joint

Larynx

Esophagus

Trachea

Shoulder joint

Elbow joint

Antebrachiocarpal joint

Middle carpal joint

Carpometacarpal joint

Metacarpophalangeal joints

Proximal interphalangeal joints

Distal interphalangeal joints

Longissimus cervicis m.

1st thoracic vertebra

Costovertebral joints

Left lung

Stomach

Spleen

15th thoracic vertebra

1st lumbar vertebra

Spiral loop of ascending colon

Left kidney

6th lumbar vertebra

Fat

Coxal tuber

Sacroiliac joint

Sacrum

1st caudal vertebra

Ilium

Rectum

Vagina

Vulva

Coxal (hip) joint

Ischiatic tuber

Ischium

Pubis

Urinary bladder

Stifle joint:
• Femoropatellar j.
• Femorotibial j.

Hock joints:
• Tarsocrural j.
• Intertarsal joints
• Tarsometatarsal j.

Metatarsophalangeal joints (fetlock joints)

Heart

Thymus

Liver

Costal cartilages

Jejunum

Apex of cecum

**PLATE 6.8**   Deep cervical muscles, major joints, and *in situ* viscera of the sow. Left lateral view. m = muscle, j = joint

**117**

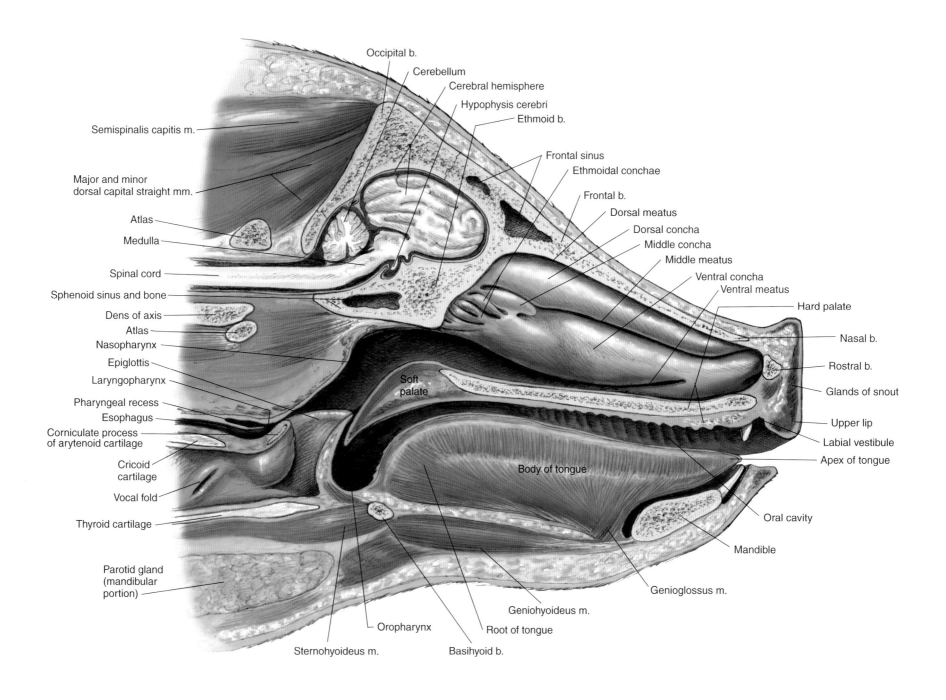

Occipital b.

Cerebellum

Cerebral hemisphere

Hypophysis cerebri

Ethmoid b.

Semispinalis capitis m.

Frontal sinus

Ethmoidal conchae

Frontal b.

Dorsal meatus

Major and minor
dorsal capital straight mm.

Dorsal concha

Middle concha

Middle meatus

Atlas

Ventral concha

Medulla

Ventral meatus

Spinal cord

Hard palate

Sphenoid sinus and bone

Nasal b.

Dens of axis

Atlas

Rostral b.

Nasopharynx

Glands of snout

Epiglottis

Soft
palate

Laryngopharynx

Upper lip

Pharyngeal recess

Labial vestibule

Esophagus

Apex of tongue

Corniculate process
of arytenoid cartilage

Body of tongue

Cricoid
cartilage

Vocal fold

Oral cavity

Thyroid cartilage

Mandible

Parotid gland
(mandibular
portion)

Geniohyoideus m.

Genioglossus m.

Oropharynx

Root of tongue

Sternohyoideus m.

Basihyoid b.

118

PLATE 6.9   Median section of the porcine head.  The nasal septum has been removed.
Right lateral view. m = muscle, b = bone

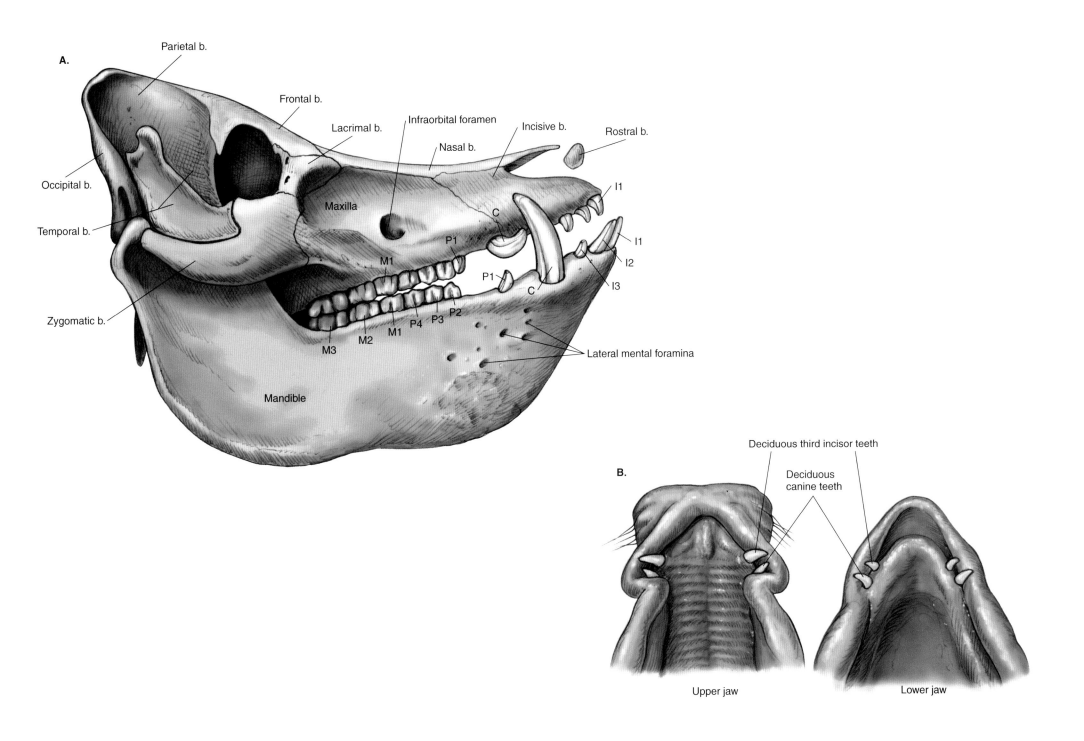

**A.** Parietal b.

Frontal b.

Lacrimal b.

Infraorbital foramen

Incisive b.

Nasal b.

Rostral b.

Occipital b.

Temporal b.

Maxilla

I1

C

Zygomatic b.

P1

I1

M1

I2

P1

I3

C

P4  P3  P2

M2  M1

M3

Mandible

Lateral mental foramina

Deciduous third incisor teeth

**B.**

Deciduous canine teeth

Upper jaw

Lower jaw

**PLATE 6.10    A.** Permanent dentition of the boar.  b = bone, I = incisor tooth,  C = canine tooth,
P = premolar tooth,  M = molar tooth  **B.** Cutting the deciduous incisor and canine teeth
of a piglet.  They are routinely cut off to prevent damage to sow's teats.

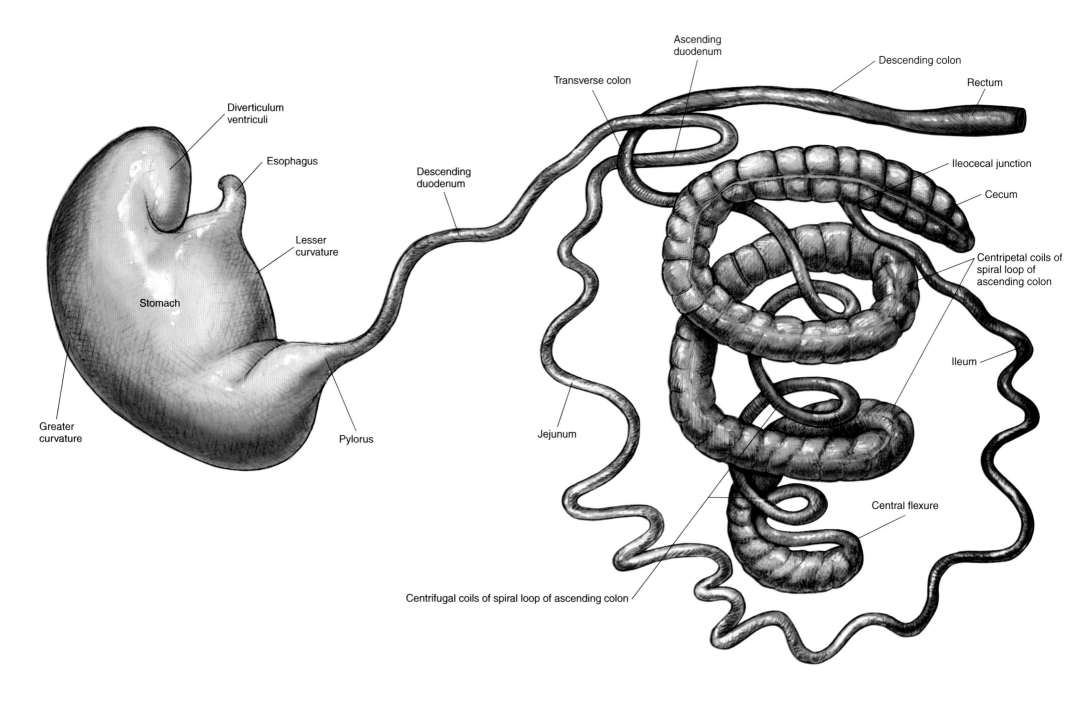

Diverticulum
ventriculi

Esophagus

Lesser
curvature

Stomach

Greater
curvature

Pylorus

Descending
duodenum

Ascending
duodenum

Transverse colon

Descending colon

Rectum

Ileocecal junction

Cecum

Centripetal coils of
spiral loop of
ascending colon

Ileum

Central flexure

Jejunum

Centrifugal coils of spiral loop of ascending colon

120

**PLATE 6.11**  Isolated stomach and intestines of the swine.  The jejunum is shortened
and uncoiled, and the loops of the ascending colon are pulled apart.

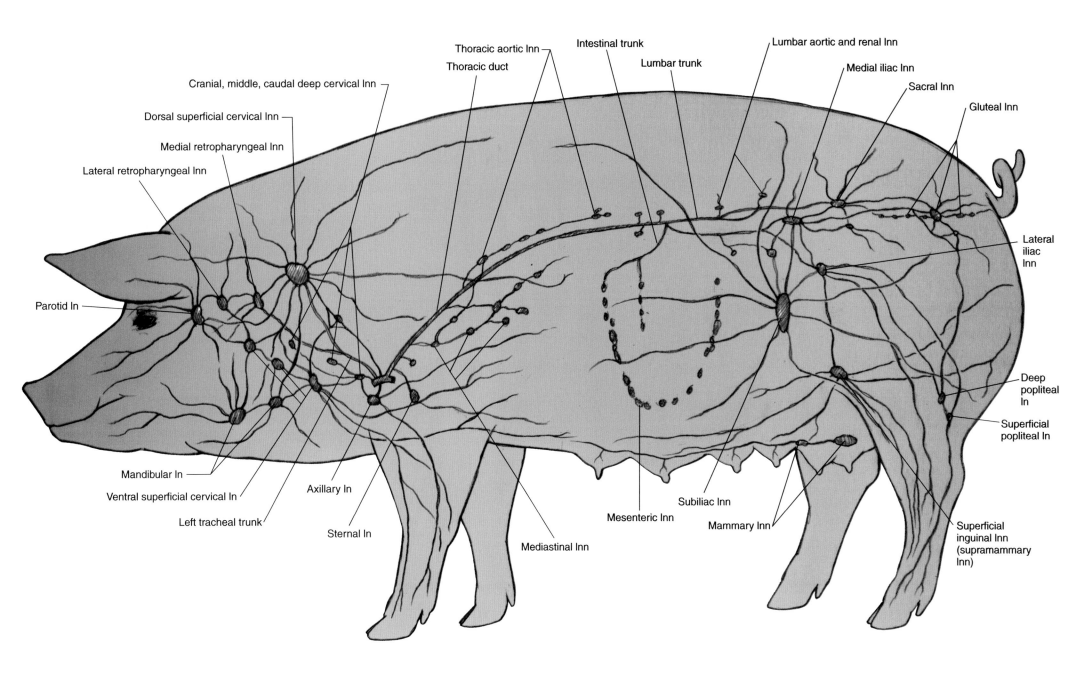

**PLATE 6.12**   Lymph nodes and vessels of the sow.   ln = lymph node

121

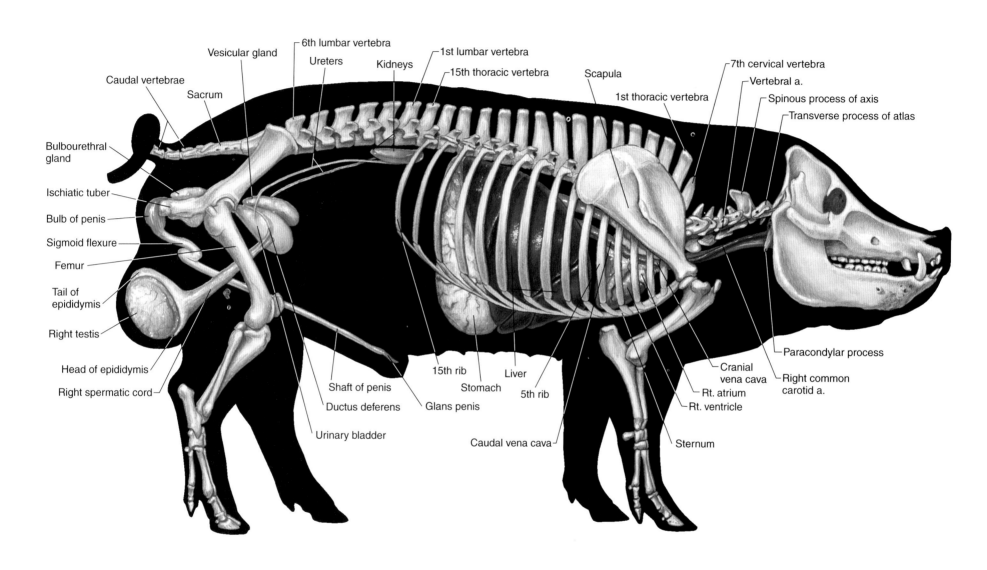

**PLATE 6.13**  Reproductive and urinary organs, stomach, liver, heart, and adjacent major vessels related to the skeleton of the boar.  Lungs and intestines are removed.  Right lateral view. a = artery

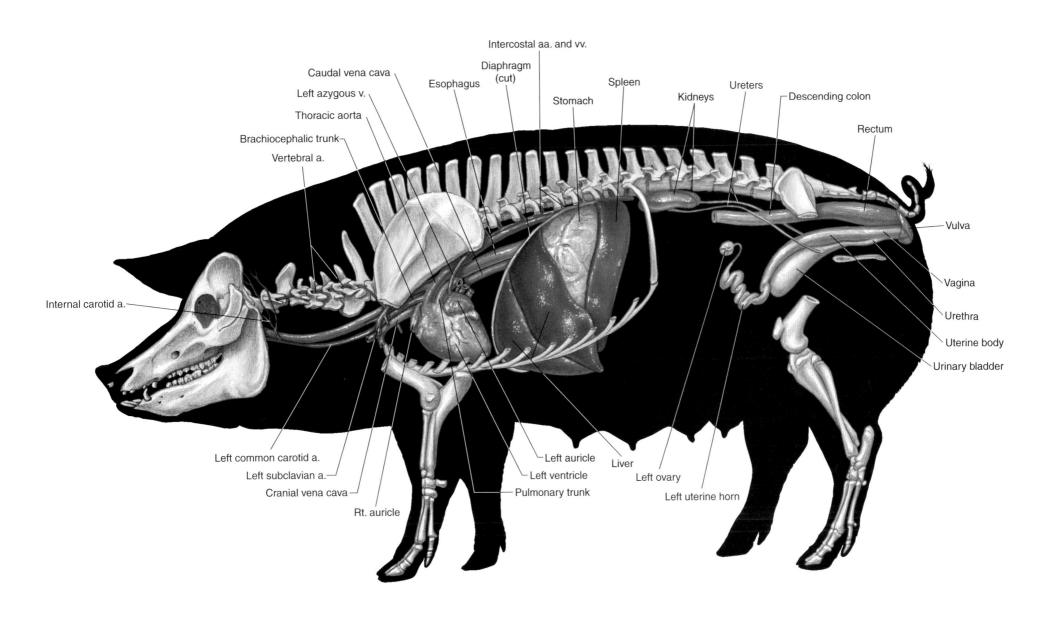

**PLATE 6.14** Reproductive and urinary organs, abdominal viscera, spleen, heart, and adjacent major vessels of the sow. Lungs and intestines are removed.
Left lateral view. v = vein, a = artery

**123**

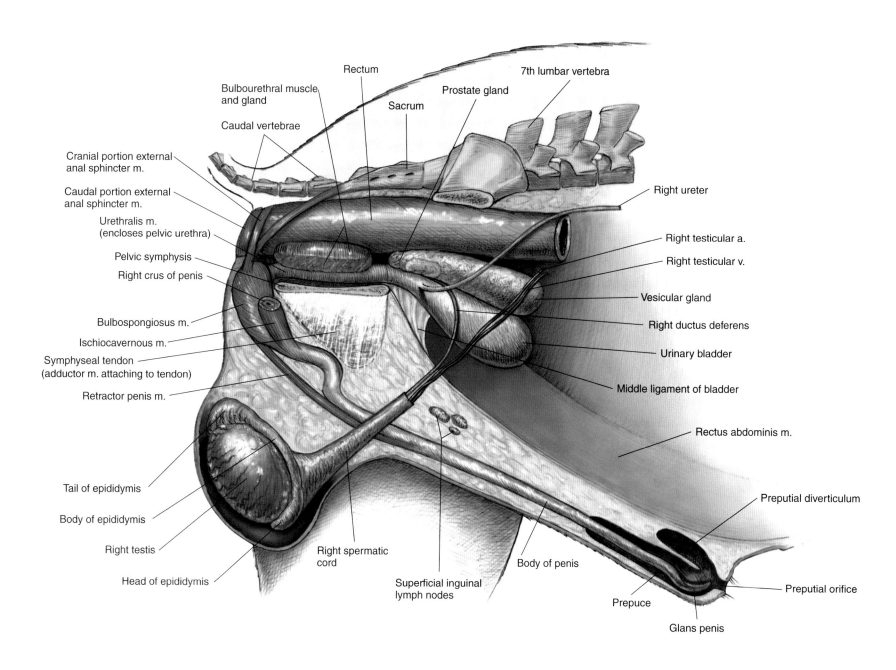

Rectum

7th lumbar vertebra

Bulbourethral muscle and gland

Prostate gland

Sacrum

Caudal vertebrae

Cranial portion external anal sphincter m.

Right ureter

Caudal portion external anal sphincter m.

Right testicular a.

Urethralis m. (encloses pelvic urethra)

Right testicular v.

Pelvic symphysis

Vesicular gland

Right crus of penis

Right ductus deferens

Bulbospongiosus m.

Urinary bladder

Ischiocavernous m.

Symphyseal tendon (adductor m. attaching to tendon)

Middle ligament of bladder

Retractor penis m.

Tail of epididymis

Rectus abdominis m.

Body of epididymis

Right testis

Preputial diverticulum

Head of epididymis

Right spermatic cord

Body of penis

Superficial inguinal lymph nodes

Preputial orifice

Prepuce

Glans penis

**PLATE 6.15**   Relations of the reproductive organs of the boar. m = muscle, v = vein, a = artery

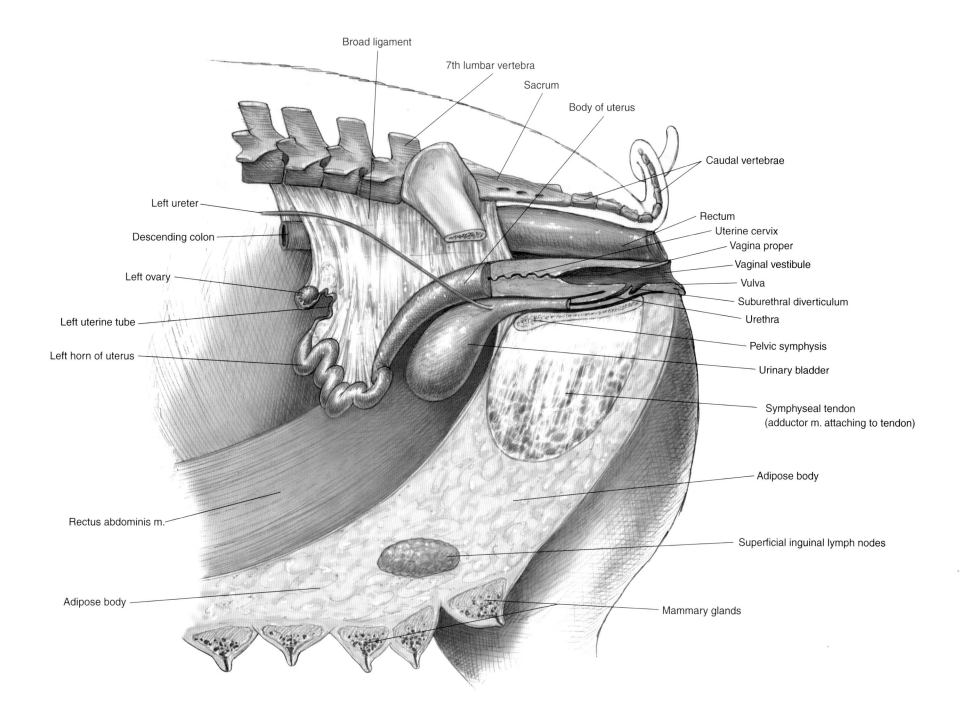

Broad ligament

7th lumbar vertebra

Sacrum

Body of uterus

Caudal vertebrae

Left ureter

Descending colon

Left ovary

Left uterine tube

Left horn of uterus

Rectum

Uterine cervix

Vagina proper

Vaginal vestibule

Vulva

Suburethral diverticulum

Urethra

Pelvic symphysis

Urinary bladder

Symphyseal tendon
(adductor m. attaching to tendon)

Adipose body

Rectus abdominis m.

Superficial inguinal lymph nodes

Adipose body

Mammary glands

**PLATE 6.16**   Relations of the reproductive organs of the sow.

# SECTION 7 THE CHICKEN
## (*Gallus gallus domesticus*)

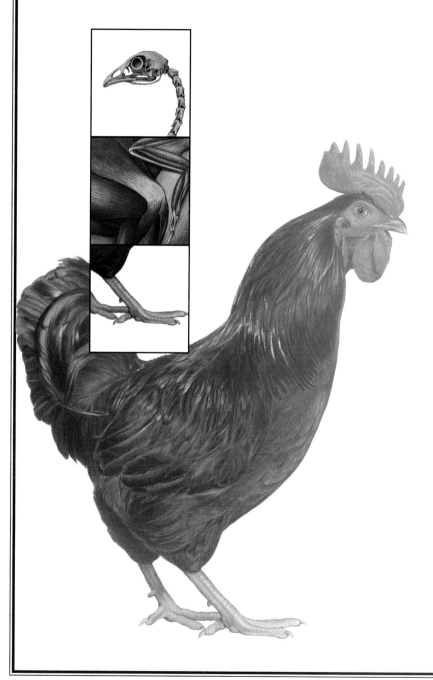

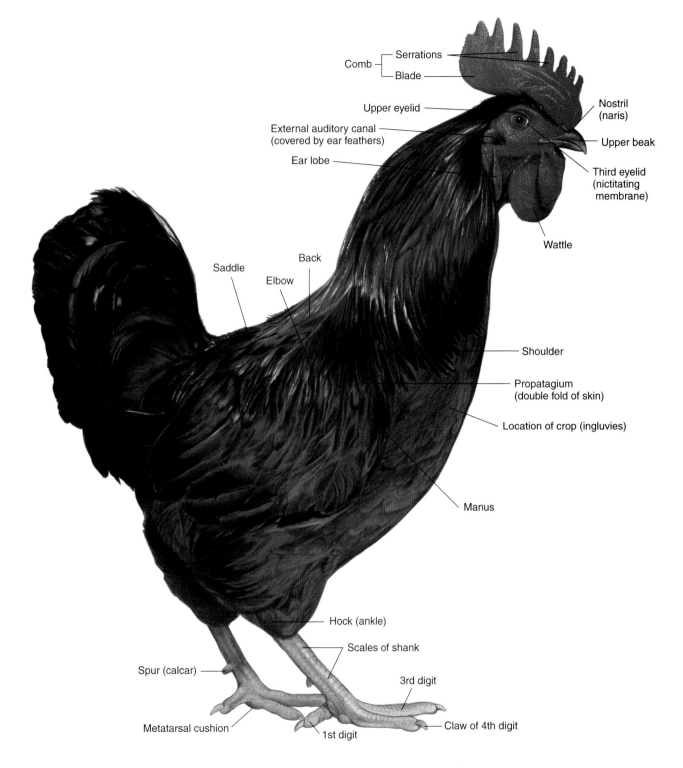

**PLATE 7.1** Right lateral view of a rooster (cock).

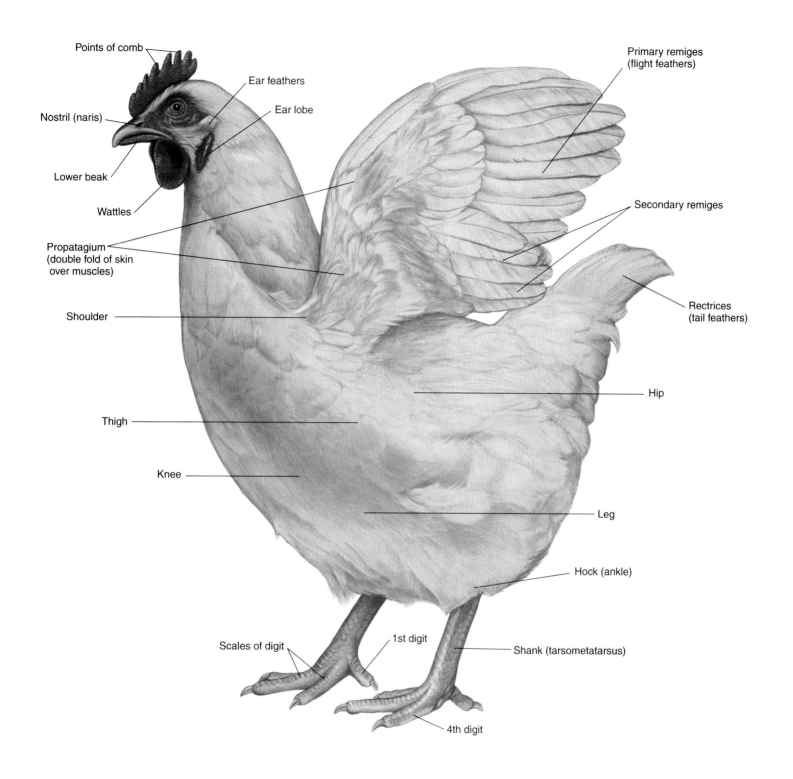

Points of comb

Ear feathers

Nostril (naris)

Ear lobe

Lower beak

Wattles

Propatagium
(double fold of skin
over muscles)

Shoulder

Thigh

Knee

Primary remiges
(flight feathers)

Secondary remiges

Rectrices
(tail feathers)

Hip

Leg

Hock (ankle)

Scales of digit

1st digit

Shank (tarsometatarsus)

4th digit

**PLATE 7.2**   Left lateral view of a hen. Patagiectomy (wing clipping), excision of part of
the propatagium (wing membrane), is performed on one wing to prevent flight.

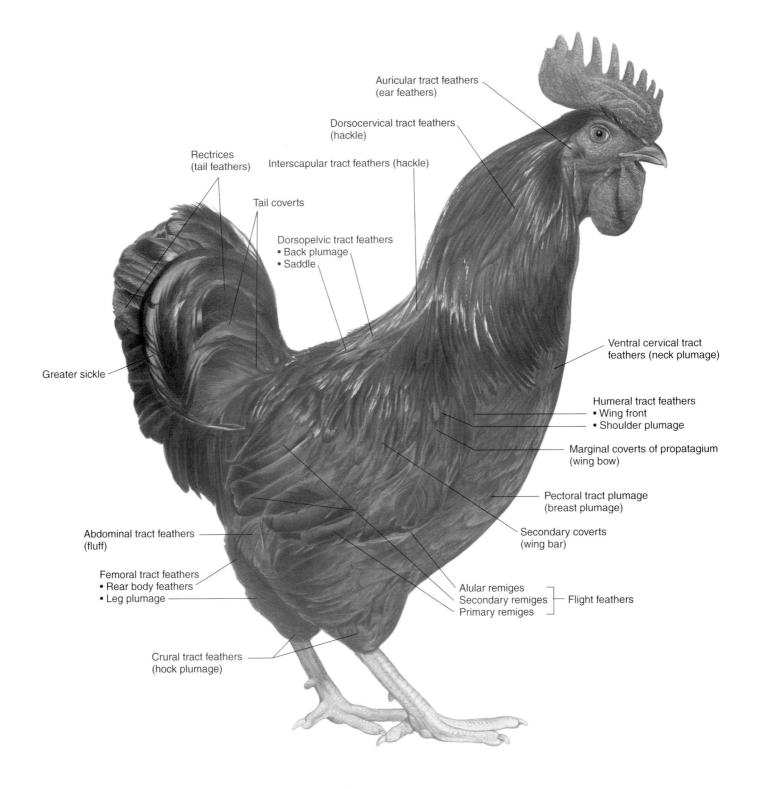

Auricular tract feathers
(ear feathers)

Dorsocervical tract feathers
(hackle)

Interscapular tract feathers (hackle)

Rectrices
(tail feathers)

Tail coverts

Dorsopelvic tract feathers
• Back plumage
• Saddle

Ventral cervical tract
feathers (neck plumage)

Greater sickle

Humeral tract feathers
• Wing front
• Shoulder plumage

Marginal coverts of propatagium
(wing bow)

Pectoral tract plumage
(breast plumage)

Abdominal tract feathers
(fluff)

Secondary coverts
(wing bar)

Femoral tract feathers
• Rear body feathers
• Leg plumage

Alular remiges
Secondary remiges      Flight feathers
Primary remiges

Crural tract feathers
(hock plumage)

130

**PLATE 7.3**   Feather coat of the rooster.

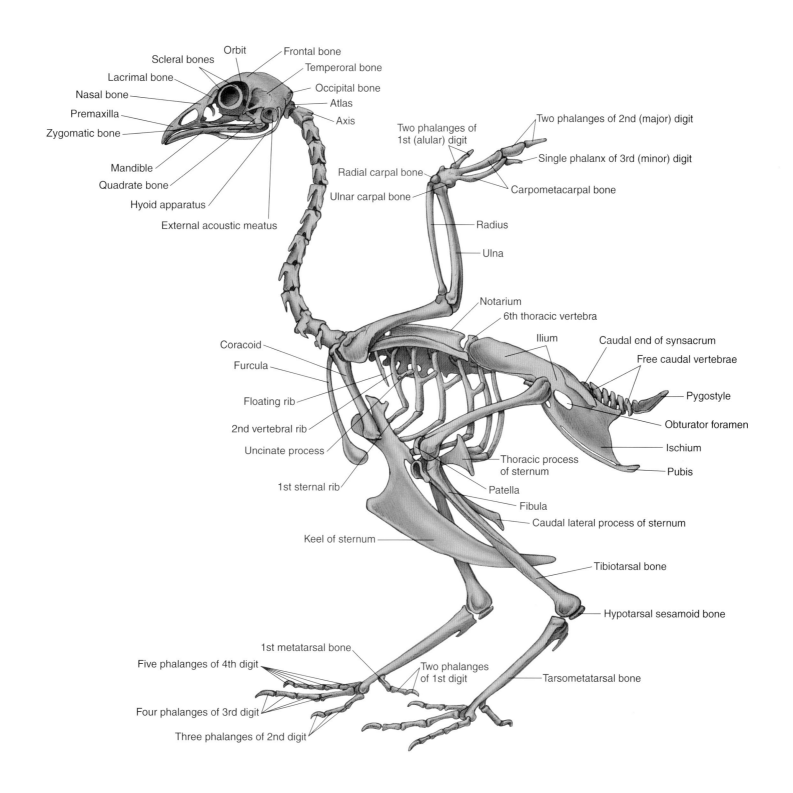

Orbit
Scleral bones
Frontal bone
Lacrimal bone
Temperoral bone
Nasal bone
Occipital bone
Premaxilla
Atlas
Zygomatic bone
Axis

Mandible
Quadrate bone
Hyoid apparatus
External acoustic meatus

Two phalanges of 1st (alular) digit
Two phalanges of 2nd (major) digit
Radial carpal bone
Single phalanx of 3rd (minor) digit
Ulnar carpal bone
Carpometacarpal bone

Radius

Ulna

Notarium
6th thoracic vertebra
Ilium
Caudal end of synsacrum
Coracoid
Free caudal vertebrae
Furcula
Pygostyle
Floating rib
2nd vertebral rib
Obturator foramen
Uncinate process
Ischium
Thoracic process of sternum
Pubis
1st sternal rib
Patella
Fibula
Caudal lateral process of sternum
Keel of sternum

Tibiotarsal bone

Hypotarsal sesamoid bone

1st metatarsal bone
Five phalanges of 4th digit
Two phalanges of 1st digit
Tarsometatarsal bone
Four phalanges of 3rd digit
Three phalanges of 2nd digit

131

**PLATE 7.4**   Skeleton of the chicken. Left lateral view.

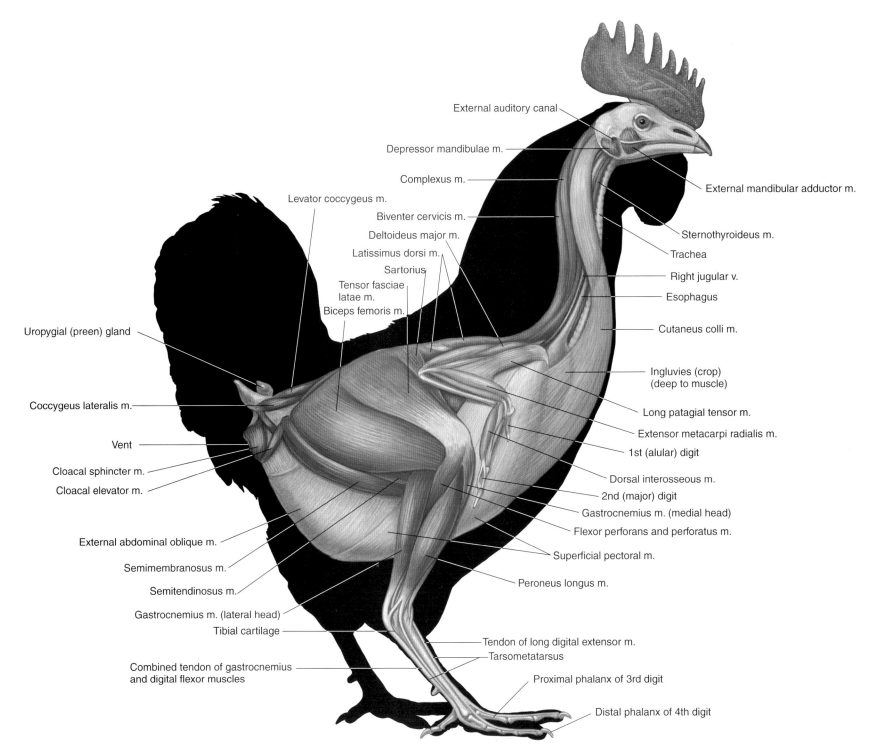

External auditory canal

Depressor mandibulae m.

Complexus m.

Levator coccygeus m.

Biventer cervicis m.

Deltoideus major m.

Latissimus dorsi m.

Sartorius

Tensor fasciae latae m.

Biceps femoris m.

External mandibular adductor m.

Sternothyroideus m.

Trachea

Right jugular v.

Esophagus

Cutaneus colli m.

Uropygial (preen) gland

Ingluvies (crop) (deep to muscle)

Long patagial tensor m.

Extensor metacarpi radialis m.

1st (alular) digit

Coccygeus lateralis m.

Vent

Cloacal sphincter m.

Cloacal elevator m.

Dorsal interosseous m.

2nd (major) digit

Gastrocnemius m. (medial head)

Flexor perforans and perforatus m.

Superficial pectoral m.

External abdominal oblique m.

Semimembranosus m.

Semitendinosus m.

Peroneus longus m.

Gastrocnemius m. (lateral head)

Tibial cartilage

Tendon of long digital extensor m.

Tarsometatarsus

Combined tendon of gastrocnemius and digital flexor muscles

Proximal phalanx of 3rd digit

Distal phalanx of 4th digit

**PLATE 7.5** Superficial muscles of the rooster. Right lateral view. m = muscle, v = vein

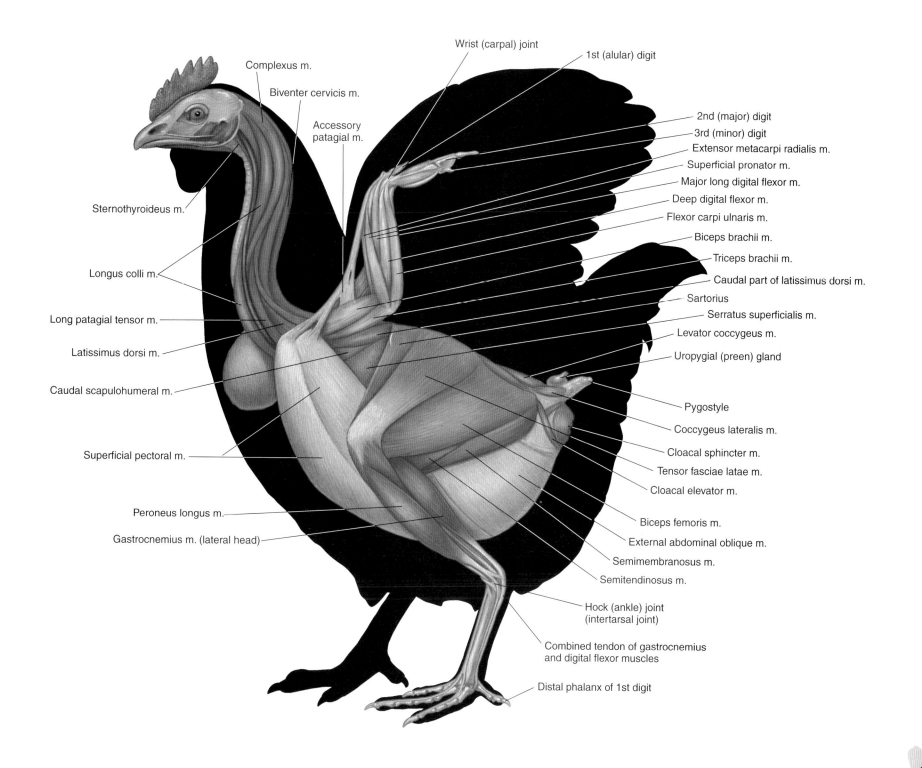

Wrist (carpal) joint

1st (alular) digit

Complexus m.

Biventer cervicis m.

Accessory
patagial m.

2nd (major) digit

3rd (minor) digit

Extensor metacarpi radialis m.

Superficial pronator m.

Major long digital flexor m.

Deep digital flexor m.

Flexor carpi ulnaris m.

Biceps brachii m.

Triceps brachii m.

Caudal part of latissimus dorsi m.

Sartorius

Serratus superficialis m.

Levator coccygeus m.

Uropygial (preen) gland

Pygostyle

Coccygeus lateralis m.

Cloacal sphincter m.

Tensor fasciae latae m.

Cloacal elevator m.

Biceps femoris m.

External abdominal oblique m.

Semimembranosus m.

Semitendinosus m.

Hock (ankle) joint
(intertarsal joint)

Combined tendon of gastrocnemius
and digital flexor muscles

Distal phalanx of 1st digit

Sternothyroideus m.

Longus colli m.

Long patagial tensor m.

Latissimus dorsi m.

Caudal scapulohumeral m.

Superficial pectoral m.

Peroneus longus m.

Gastrocnemius m. (lateral head)

**133**

**PLATE 7.6**  Superficial muscles of the hen. Left lateral view. m = muscle

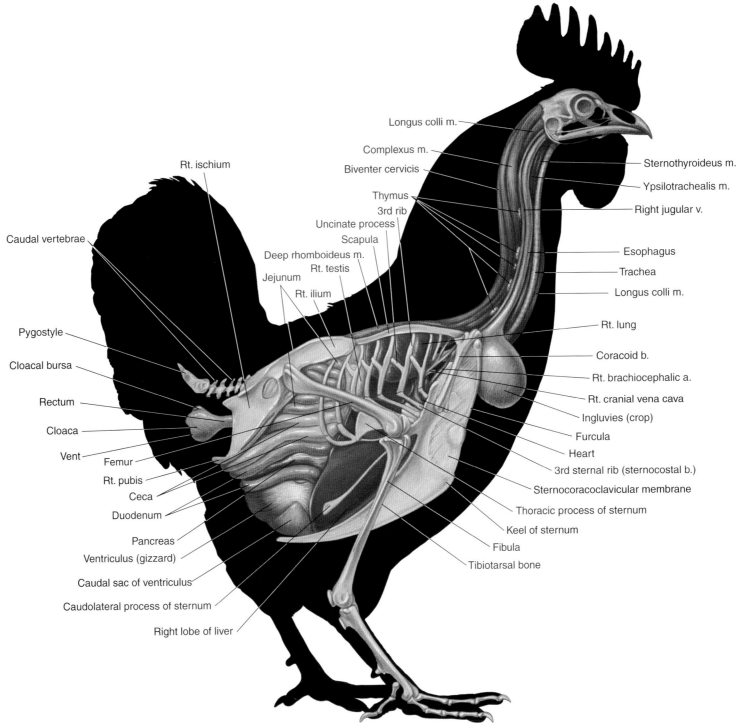

Longus colli m.

Complexus m.

Biventer cervicis

Sternothyroideus m.

Ypsilotrachealis m.

Thymus

3rd rib

Right jugular v.

Uncinate process

Scapula

Esophagus

Rt. ischium

Deep rhomboideus m.

Trachea

Rt. testis

Jejunum

Longus colli m.

Caudal vertebrae

Rt. ilium

Rt. lung

Pygostyle

Coracoid b.

Rt. brachiocephalic a.

Cloacal bursa

Rt. cranial vena cava

Rectum

Ingluvies (crop)

Furcula

Cloaca

Heart

Vent

3rd sternal rib (sternocostal b.)

Femur

Sternocoracoclavicular membrane

Rt. pubis

Thoracic process of sternum

Ceca

Keel of sternum

Duodenum

Fibula

Pancreas

Tibiotarsal bone

Ventriculus (gizzard)

Caudal sac of ventriculus

Caudolateral process of sternum

Right lobe of liver

134

**PLATE 7.7**   Relations of *in situ* viscera to the skeleton and cervical muscles of the rooster.
Right lateral view. m = muscle, b = bone, a = artery, v = vein

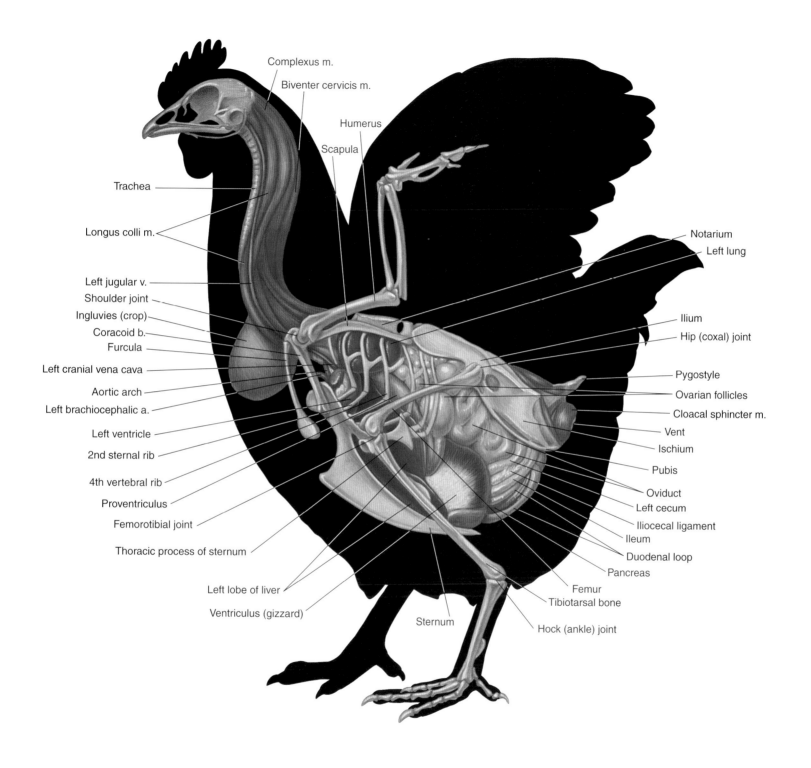

Complexus m.

Biventer cervicis m.

Humerus

Scapula

Trachea

Longus colli m.

Notarium

Left lung

Left jugular v.

Shoulder joint

Ingluvies (crop)

Coracoid b.

Furcula

Left cranial vena cava

Aortic arch

Left brachiocephalic a.

Left ventricle

2nd sternal rib

4th vertebral rib

Proventriculus

Femorotibial joint

Thoracic process of sternum

Ilium

Hip (coxal) joint

Pygostyle

Ovarian follicles

Cloacal sphincter m.

Vent

Ischium

Pubis

Oviduct

Left cecum

Iliocecal ligament

Ileum

Duodenal loop

Pancreas

Femur

Tibiotarsal bone

Left lobe of liver

Ventriculus (gizzard)

Sternum

Hock (ankle) joint

**PLATE 7.8** Relations of *in situ* viscera and blood vessels to the skeleton and cervical muscles of the hen. Left lateral view. m = muscle, v = vein, b = bone, a = artery

135

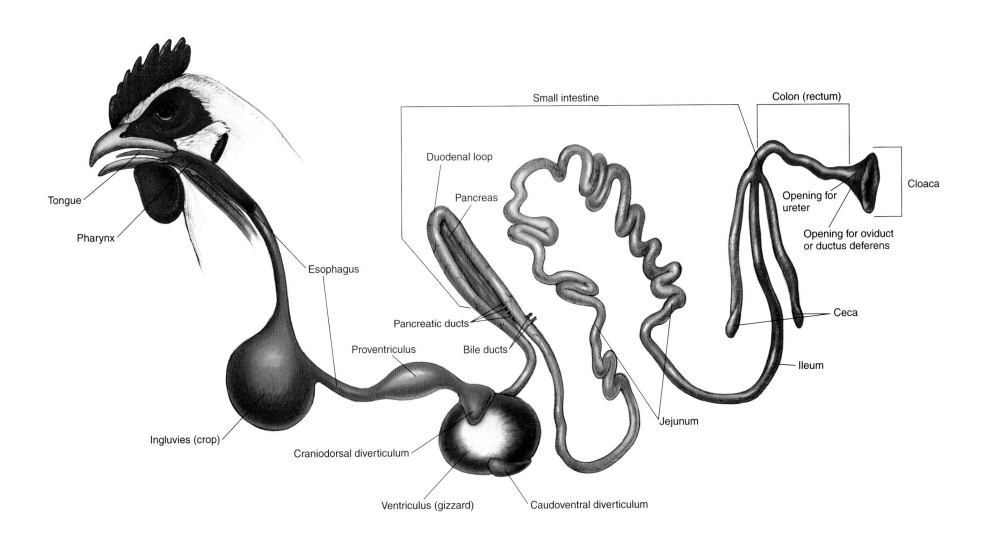

**PLATE 7.9**    Isolated gastrointestinal tract of the chicken.

**136**

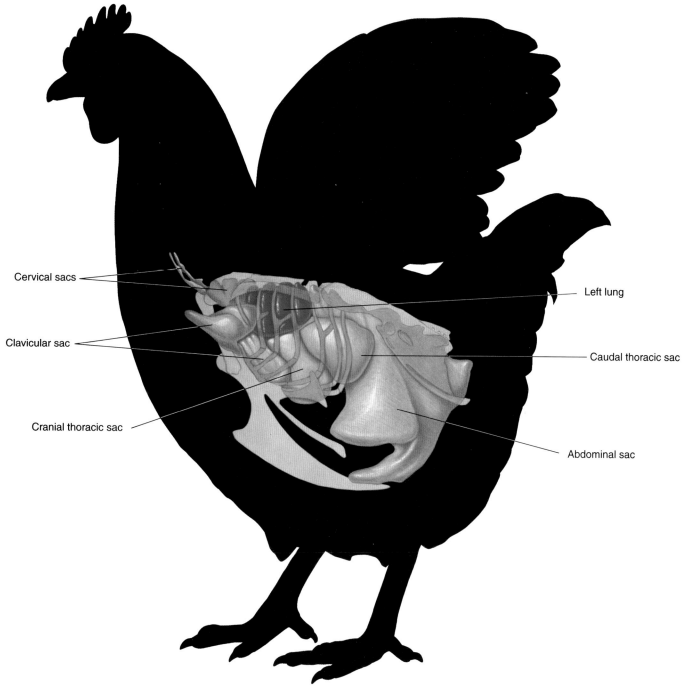

Cervical sacs

Clavicular sac

Cranial thoracic sac

Left lung

Caudal thoracic sac

Abdominal sac

**PLATE 7.10** Air sacs and lungs of the chicken. Left lateral view. There is a total of eleven air sacs named according to location: abdominal, caudal thoracic, cranial thoracic, axillary, clavicular, and cervical. All are paired except the single clavicular sac. With the exception of the thoracic sacs, all provide communication between a bronchus and the interior of some of the pneumatic (air-containing) bones.

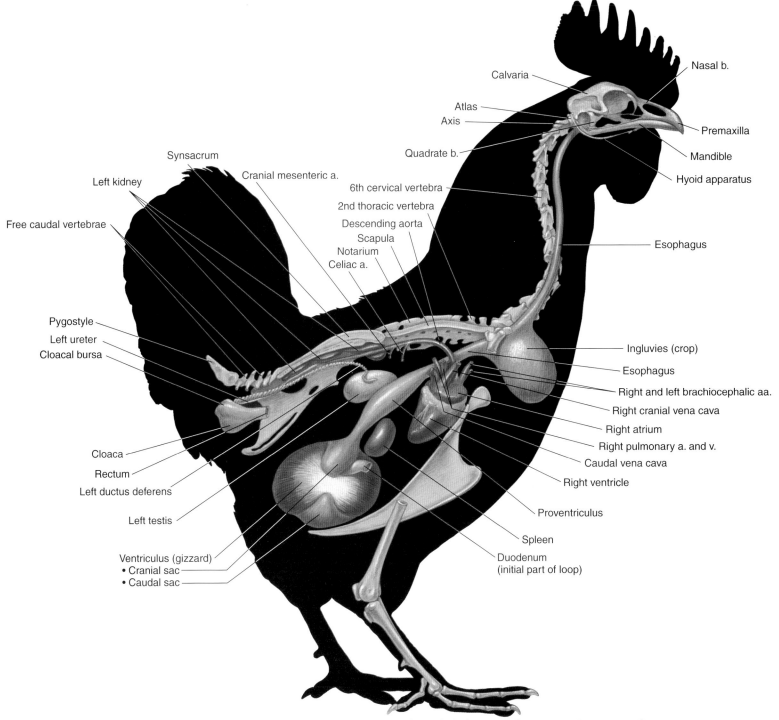

Calvaria

Nasal b.

Atlas

Axis

Premaxilla

Quadrate b.

Mandible

Synsacrum

Cranial mesenteric a.

6th cervical vertebra

Hyoid apparatus

Left kidney

2nd thoracic vertebra

Descending aorta

Free caudal vertebrae

Scapula

Esophagus

Notarium

Celiac a.

Pygostyle

Ingluvies (crop)

Left ureter

Esophagus

Cloacal bursa

Right and left brachiocephalic aa.

Right cranial vena cava

Right atrium

Right pulmonary a. and v.

Caudal vena cava

Cloaca

Right ventricle

Rectum

Left ductus deferens

Proventriculus

Left testis

Spleen

Ventriculus (gizzard)

• Cranial sac

Duodenum
(initial part of loop)

• Caudal sac

138

**PLATE 7.11** *In situ* viscera, major blood vessels, and axial skeleton of the rooster. Intestines, liver, and lungs are removed. Right lateral view. b = bone, a = artery, v = vein

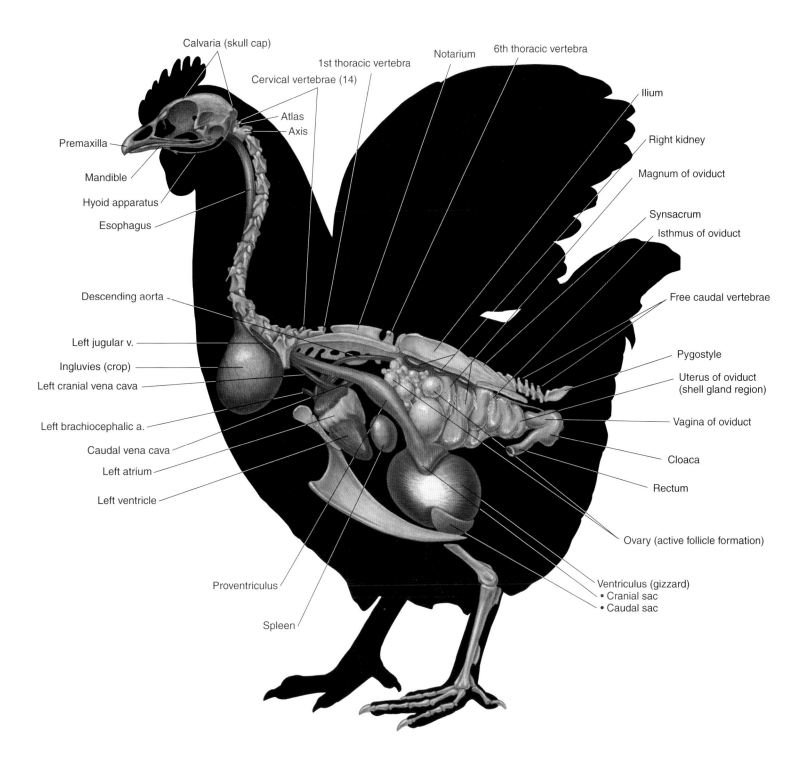

Calvaria (skull cap)

1st thoracic vertebra

Notarium

6th thoracic vertebra

Cervical vertebrae (14)

Ilium

Atlas

Axis

Premaxilla

Right kidney

Mandible

Magnum of oviduct

Hyoid apparatus

Synsacrum

Esophagus

Isthmus of oviduct

Descending aorta

Free caudal vertebrae

Left jugular v.

Ingluvies (crop)

Pygostyle

Left cranial vena cava

Uterus of oviduct
(shell gland region)

Left brachiocephalic a.

Vagina of oviduct

Caudal vena cava

Cloaca

Left atrium

Rectum

Left ventricle

Ovary (active follicle formation)

Proventriculus

Ventriculus (gizzard)
• Cranial sac
• Caudal sac

Spleen

**139**

**PLATE 7.12** *In situ* viscera, major blood vessels, and axial skeleton of the hen. Intestines, liver, and lungs are removed. Left lateral view. v = vein, a = artery

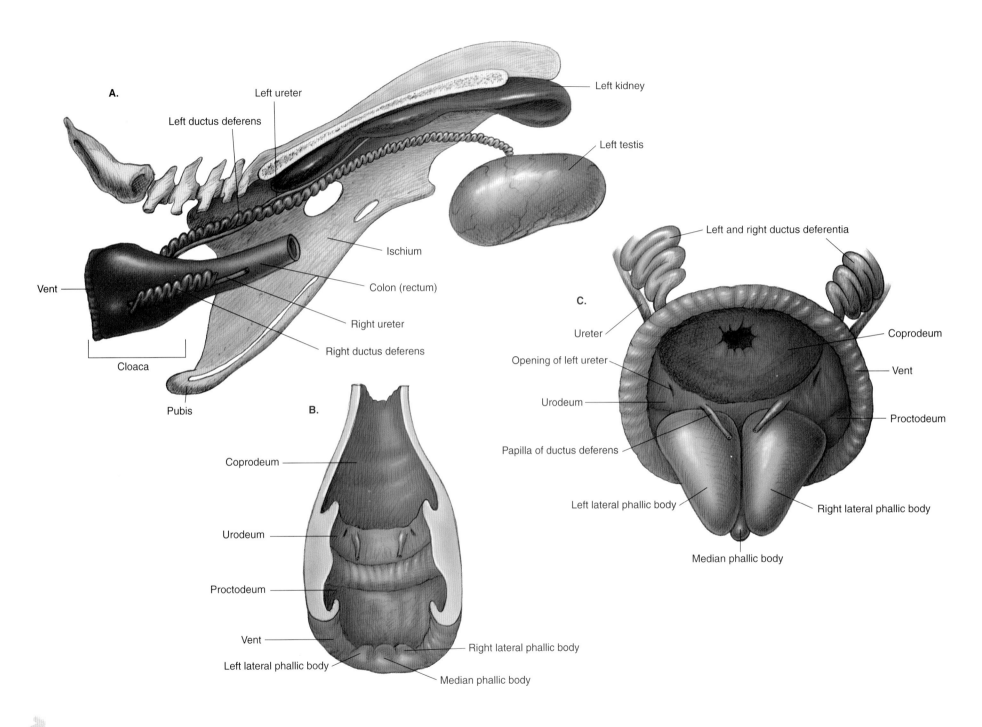

A. Reproductive and urinary organs of the rooster. Right lateral view.

**A.**

Left ureter

Left ductus deferens

Left kidney

Left testis

Ischium

Colon (rectum)

Vent

Right ureter

Right ductus deferens

Cloaca

Pubis

**B.**

Coprodeum

Urodeum

Proctodeum

Vent

Left lateral phallic body

Right lateral phallic body

Median phallic body

**C.**

Left and right ductus deferentia

Ureter

Opening of left ureter

Urodeum

Papilla of ductus deferens

Left lateral phallic body

Coprodeum

Vent

Proctodeum

Right lateral phallic body

Median phallic body

140

**PLATE 7. 13   A.** Reproductive and urinary organs of the rooster. Right lateral view. **B.** Cloaca of the rooster. Dorsal view. **C.** Erect copulatory apparatus. Caudodorsal view.

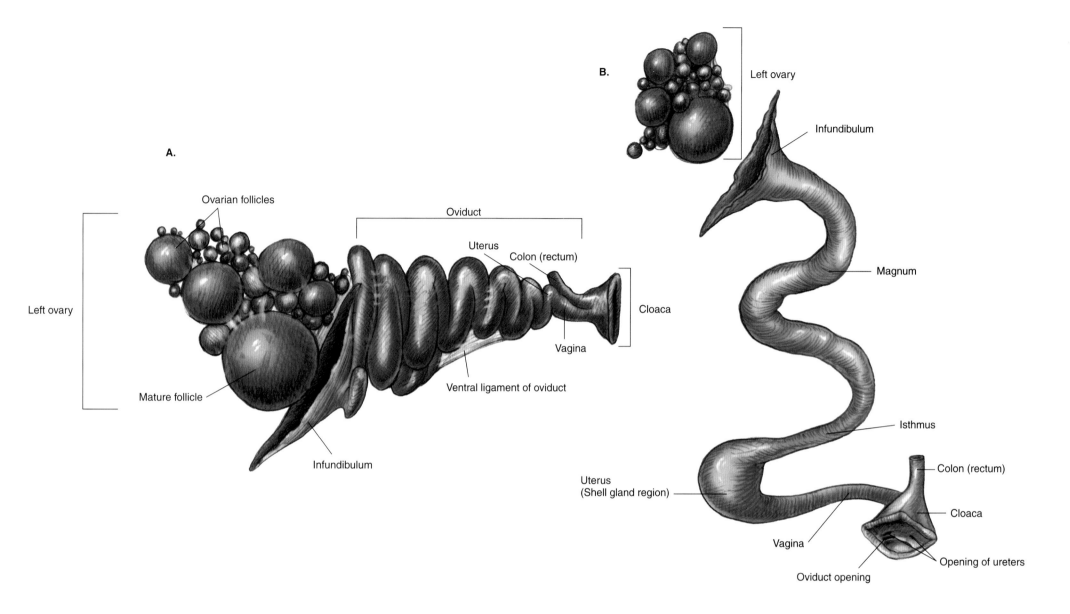

**A.**

Ovarian follicles

Left ovary

Mature follicle

Infundibulum

Oviduct

Uterus

Colon (rectum)

Cloaca

Vagina

Ventral ligament of oviduct

**B.**

Left ovary

Infundibulum

Magnum

Isthmus

Colon (rectum)

Cloaca

Uterus
(Shell gland region)

Vagina

Oviduct opening

Opening of ureters

**141**

**PLATE 7. 14   A.** Isolated reproductive organs of the hen. Left lateral view.
**B.** Diagrammatic representation of the reproductive organs of the hen.

# BIBLIOGRAPHY

Ashdown PR, Done SH. Color Atlas of Veterinary Anatomy—The Ruminants. London: Bailliere Tindall, 1984.

Ashdown PR, Done SH. Color Atlas of Veterinary Anatomy—The Horse. London: Bailliere Tindall, 1987.

Budras K-D, Sack WO, Rock S. Anatomy of the Horse—An Illustrated Text. London: Mosby-Wolfe, 1994.

Chamberlain F. Atlas of Avian Anatomy. East Lansing, Michigan: State College Press, 1943.

Clayton HM, Flood PF. Color Atlas of Large Animal Applied Anatomy. London: Mosby-Wolfe, 1996.

de Lahunta A, Habel RE. Applied Veterinary Anatomy. Philadelphia: WB Saunders, 1986.

Dyce KM, Sack WO, Wensing GJG. Textbook of Veterinary Anatomy. Philadelphia: WB Saunders, 1987.

Ellenberger W. Leisering's Atlas of Anatomy, Vol 1. Chicago: Alexander Eger, 1908.

Ellenberger W, Dittrich H, Baum HM. An Atlas of Animal Anatomy. London: Dover, 1949.

Ellenberger W, Baum HM. Handbuch der Vergleichenden Anatomie der Haustiere. 18th ed. Berlin: Springer, 1977.

Fowler ME. Medicine and Surgery of South American Camelids: Llama, Alpaca, Vicuna, Guanaco. Ames, IA: Iowa State University Press, 1995.

Garrett PD. Guide to Ruminant Anatomy Based on the Dissection of the Goat. Ames, IA: Iowa State University Press, 1988.

Gertty R. Sisson and Grossman's The Anatomy of the Domestic Animals, 5th ed, Vols I and II. Philadelphia: WB Saunders, 1975.

Goshal NG, Koch T, Popesko P. The Venous Drainage of the Domestic Animals. Philadelphia: WB Saunders, 1981.

Harvey EB, Kaiser HE, Rosenberg LE. An Atlas of the Domestic Turkey. United States Atomic Energy Commission, 1948.

Kainer RA. Functional anatomy of equine locomotor organs. In: Stashak T, ed. Adams' Lameness in Horses. 5th ed. Philadelphia: Lippincott Williams & Wilkins, 1999.

Kainer RA, McCracken TO. Horse Anatomy—A Coloring Atlas. 2nd ed. Loveland, CO: Alpine Publications, 1998.

McLeod WM, Trotter DM, Lumb JW. Avian Anatomy. Minneapolis: Burgess Publishing Co, 1964.

The Meat Buyers Guide. National Association of Meat Purveyors, McLean, VA, 1992.

Moreng RE, Avens JS. Poultry Science and Production. Prospect Heights, IL: Waveland Press, 1981.

Nickel R, Schummer A, Seiferle E, et al. The Locomotor System of the Domestic Animals, Vol 1. Berlin-Hamburg: Paul Parey, 1986.

Nickel R, Schummer A, Seiferle E. Nervensystem. Sinnesorgane und Endokrine Drusen, Vol 4. Berlin-Hamburg: Paul Parey, 1992.

Nickel R, Schummer A, Seiferle E. Anatomy of the Domestic Birds, Vol 5. Berlin-Hamburg: Paul Parey, 1977.

Pfizer Animal Health Group. Anatomical Atlas. New York: Pfizer Corporation, 1976.

Popesko P. Atlas of Topographic Anatomy of the Domestic Animals. Philadelphia: WB Saunders, 1979.

Sack WO, Habel RE. Rooney's Guide to the Dissection of the Horse. Ithaca, NY: Veterinary Textbooks, 1977.

Sack WO, Horowitz A. Essentials of Pig Anatomy & Atlas of Musculoskeletal Anatomy of the Pig. Ithaca, NY: Veterinary Textbooks, 1982.

Schummer A, Nickel R, Sack WO. The Viscera of the Domestic Animals, Vol 2. Berlin-Hamburg: Paul Parey, 1979.

Schummer A, Wilkins H, Vollmerhaus B, Habermehl K-H. The Circulatory System, the Skin, and the Cutaneous Organs of the Domestic Animals, Vol 3. Berlin-Hamburg: Paul Parey, 1981.

Senger PL. Pathways to Pregnancy and Parturition. Pullman, WA: Senger, 1997.

Shively MJ. Veterinary Anatomy—Basic, Comparative and Clinical. College Station, TX: Texas A & M University, 1984.

Smallwood JE. A Guided Tour of Veterinary Anatomy. Philadelphia: WB Saunders, 1992.

# INDEX

References to the various animals described in this atlas are indicated by the following letters preceding page numbers: **H,** horse; **O,** ox; **S,** sheep; **G,** goat; **L,** llama and alpaca; **Sw,** swine; **C,** chicken.

## A

Abdomen, **L** 90; **Sw** 111
Abdominal tunic, **O** 37
Abomasum, **O** 38, 42, 43, 45; **S** 60, 61, 64, 65; **G** 80, 81, 84
Adipose body, **Sw** 125
Air sacs, **C** 137
Ankle, **H** 2 (fetlock); **C** 128, 129 (hock)
Antebrachium, **H** 2; **O** 33; **G** 72; **L** 90
Anus, **H** 13, 20, 22, 23; **O** 41, 45, 46, 47; **S** 67; **G** 85, 86, 87; **L** 106, 107; **Sw** 117
Aorta. *See* Artery or Arteries
Arm, **H** 2; **O** 32, 33; **S** 54; **G** 72; **L** 90
Artery or Arteries
    aorta, **H** 24, 25; **O** 44, 45, 49; **S** 64, 64; **G** 84, 85, 87; **L** 104, 105; **Sw** 123; **C** 135, 138, 139
    artery of the lateral sinus, **G** 87
    axillary, **H** 25, 49
    bicarotid trunk, **S** 65; **G** 85
    brachial, **H** 25; **O** 49
    brachiocephalic trunk, **H** 21, 25; **O** 45, 49; **S** 65; **L** 104, 105; **Sw** 123
    bronchoesophageal, **O** 49
    caudal auricular, **H** 25; **O** 49; **G** 82
    caudal epigastric, **H** 25; **O** 49; **G** 85, 87
    caudal femoral, **H** 25; **O** 49
    caudal gluteal, **H** 25; **O** 49; **G** 87
    caudal interosseous, **O** 49
    caudal mammary, **O** 49; **G** 87

    caudal meningeal, **G** 82
    caudal mesenteric, **H** 25; **O** 49
    caudal superficial epigastric, **G** 87
    caudal tibial, **H** 25; **O** 49
    celiac, **H** 25; **O** 49; **C** 138
    collateral ulnar, **H** 25; **O** 49
    common carotid, **H** 25; **O** 44, 45, 49; **S** 62, 64, 65; **G** 82, 84, 85; **L** 101, 104, 105; **Sw** 122, 123
    common interosseous, **H** 20, 21, 25; **O** 44, 45, 59; **S** 62, 64, 65; **G** 82, 84, 85
    condylar, **G** 82
    cornual, **G** 80, 82
    costocervical trunk, **H** 25
    cranial epigastric, **H** 25; **O** 49
    cranial gluteal, **H** 25; **O** 49
    cranial interosseous, **O** 49
    cranial mammary, **O** 49; **G** 87
    cranial mesenteric, **H** 25; **O** 49; **C** 138
    cranial tibial, **H** 25; **O** 49
    deep cervical, **H** 25; **O** 49
    deep circumflex iliac, **H** 25; **O** 49
    deep femoral, **H** 25; **O** 49; **G** 85, 87
    descending genicular, **H** 25
    digital, **H** 25; **G** 78; **L** 96
    distal perforating branch, **H** 25
    dorsal, **H** 25; **O** 49
    dorsal common digital, **O** 49
    dorsal metacarpal III, **O** 49
    dorsal metatarsal III, **O** 49
    dorsal nasal, **G** 82
    dorsal pedal, **H** 25; **O** 49
    dorsal proper digital, **O** 49
    ethmoid, **G** 82

Coprodeum. *See* Cloaca

Corium of foot, **H** 9; **G** 79

Cornual process, **O** 38

Coronet, **H**3

Coxal tuber. *See* Bone(s)

Crest, **H**2

Crop. *See* Ingluvies

Croup, **H** 2

Crus, **H** 2; **O** 36; **S** 55; **L** 90, 91

## D

Dental pad, **O** 40, 44; **S** 60; **G** 82, 83, 84; **L** 99

Dermis of foot. *See* Corium of foot

Dewclaws, **O** 32, 33; **G** 72, 73, 78, 79

Dewlap, **O** 33

Diaphragm, **H** 20, 21; **O** 40, 42, 43, 44, 45; **G** 84; **L** 105; **Sw** 123

Digit(s), **H** 2, 8; **O** 33, **G** 78, 79; **L** 96; **Sw** 110, 113; **C** 128, 129, 131, 132, 133

    accessory, **Sw** 110

Digital cushion, **H** 8; **G** 79

Digital pad. *See* Slipper

Digital sheath, **H** 8

Diverticulum ventriculi. *See* Stomach

Dock. *See* Tail head

Ductus deferens, **H** 20, 22; **O** 44, 46; **S** 64, 66; **G** 84, 86; **L** 104, 106; **Sw** 122, 124; **C** 136, 138, 140

    ampulla, **H** 22; **S** 66; **L** 106

    convoluted part, **H** 22

    papilla, **C** 140

Duodenum, **H** 12, 16; **O** 38, 42, 43; **S** 60, 64; **G** 80; **L** 96, 103; **Sw** 120; **C** 134, 135, 136, 138

    ampulla, **L** 103, 104

## E

Ear. *See also* Pinna

    ear feathers. *See* Feather(s)

    ear lobe, **C** 128, 129

    "flop" ear, **Sw** 110

    "prick" ear, **Sw** 111

Elbow, **C** 128

Epididymis, **H** 22; **O** 44, 46; **G** 84, 86; **L** 104, 106; **Sw** 122, 124

Epiglottis, **O** 40; **G** 83; **L** 99; **Sw** 118

Ergot, **H** 3

Esophagus, **H** 12, 13, 14, 20, 21; **O** 38, 39, 40, 41, 44; **S** 60, 61, 62, 64, 65; **G** 80, 81, 83, 84, 85; **L** 99, 101, 103, 105; **Sw** 117, 120, 123; **C** 132, 134, 136, 138, 139

External acoustic meatus. *See* Temporal bone, **H** 5, **G** 45

External auditory canal, **C** 128, 132

Eyelid

    third, **C** 128

    upper, **H** 2; **Sw** 110; **C** 128

## F

Face, **H** 2; **O** 32, 33; **S** 54; **G** 72, 73; **L** 90

Facial crest, **H** 3

Fascia

    abdominal, **O** 36; **S** 58; **G** 76; **L** 94

    antebrachial, **H** 6; **O** 36; **S** 58; **G** 76; **L** 94; **Sw** 114

    cervical, **H** 6; **L** 94

    crural, **H** 6; **O** 36; **S** 58; **G** 76; **L** 94; **Sw** 114

    fascia lata, **H** 6, 7; **O** 36; **S** 58; **G** 76; **L** 94; **Sw** 114

    femoral, **H** 6; **O** 36; **S** 58; **G** 76; **Sw** 114

    omobrachial, **G** 76

    superficial f. of trunk, **H** 6; **O** 36; **S** 58; **G** 76; **L** 94; **Sw** 114

    superficial gluteal, **H** 6; **O** 36; **S** 58; **G** 76; **L** 94; **Sw** 114

    thoracolumbar, **H** 7; **O** 37; **S** 59; **G** 77; **L** 95; **Sw** 115

Feather(s)

    covert, **C** 130

    ear, **C** 128, 129, 130

    f. tracts, **C** 130

    rectrices (tail f.), **C** 120, 130

    remiges (flight f.), **C** 129, 130

    sickle, **C** 130

    wing bar, **C** 130

    wing bow, **C** 130

Fetlock, **H** 2; **O** 32; **S** 54; **G** 72; **L** 90; **Sw** 110

Flank, **S** 56; **L** 90; **Sw** 110. *See also* Fold, flank

Flexures

    diaphragmatic f. of ascending colon, **H** 16, 17, 19

distal sesamoidean, **H** 10, 11

distal sesamoidean impar, **H** 8

dorsal l. of tarsus, **O** 37; **G** 77

interdigital, **G** 78

middle l. of bladder, **H** 24; **G** 86; **Sw** 124

nephrosplenic, **H** 19

nuchal, **H** 13, 14, 21; **O** 39, 40; **S** 61; **G** 81, 83; **L** 95, 96, 97, 99, 105

palmar anular, **H** 8

radial check, **H** 10

supraspinous, **H** 21; **O** 38, 39; **S** 61; **G** 81; **L** 96, 97

suspensory (interosseus medius m.), **H** 7, 10, 11; **O** 37; **S** 59; **G** 77; **L** 95, 98

"T", **H** 7

triangular l. of liver, **H** 21

ventral l. of oviduct, **C** 141

Linea alba, **G** 86; **L** 106

Lingual fossa. *See* Tongue

Lips, **H** 14; **O** 40; **G** 73, 83; **L** 99; **Sw** 110, 118

Liver, **H** 12, 20, 21, 24; **O** 38, 42, 43, 44; **S** 60; **G** 80, 84; **L** 96, 104; **Sw** 116, 117, 122, 123; **C** 134, 135

    caudate process of caudate lobe, **O** 44

    left lobe, **H** 21; **O** 44

    quadrate lobe, **H** 20; **O** 44

    right lobe, **H** 20; **O** 44; **L** 104

Loin, **H** 2; **O** 32; **S** 54.56; **G** 72; **L** 90; **Sw** 110, 111, 112

Lower foreshank, **S** 54, 56

Lower hindshank, **S** 54, 56

Lumbosacral plexus. *See* Nerve(s)

Lung, **H** 12, 13; **O** 38, 39, 40; **S** 60, 61; **G** 80, 81; **L** 96, 97; **Sw** 116, 117; **C** 134, 135, 137

Lymph node(s)

    axillary, **H** 27; **O** 51; **Sw** 121

    caudal deep cervical, **H** 27; **O** 51; **Sw** 121

    caudal mediastinal, **O** 45; **S** 65; **G** 84, 5

    caudal mesenteric, **H** 27

    cranial deep cervical, **H** 27, **O** 51; **Sw** 121

    deep inguinal, **H** 27

    dorsal thoracic, **H** 27

    epigastric, **O** 51

    gluteal, **O** 51; **Sw** 121

    intercostal, **O** 51

    lateral iliac, **O** 51; **Sw** 121

    lateral retropharyngeal, **H** 27; **O** 38, 51, 56; **Sw** 121

    lumbar aortic and renal, **H** 27; **O** 51; **Sw** 121

    mandibular, **H** 27; **O** 51; **S** 62; **Sw** 121

    medial iliac, **H** 27; **O** 51; **Sw** 121

    medial retropharyngeal, **H** 27; **O** 51; **Sw** 121

    mediastinal, **H** 27; **L** 104; **Sw** 121

    mesenteric, **H** 27; **O** 51; **Sw** 121

    middle deep cervical, **H** 27; **O** 51; **Sw** 121

    parotid, **H** 27; **O** 51; **Sw** 121

    popliteal, **H** 27; **O** 51; **Sw** 121

        deep, **Sw** 121

        superficial, **Sw** 121

    sacral, **H** 27; **Sw** 121

    sternal, **O** 51; **Sw** 121

    subiliac, **H** 7, 27; **O** 36, 51; **G** 77; **L** 93; **Sw** 114, 121

    superficial cervical, **H** 27; **O** 38, 51; **L** 101

        dorsal, **Sw** 121

        ventral, **Sw** 121

    superficial inguinal, **H** 27; **O** 39, 51; **S** 66, 67; **G** 81, 84; **L** 106, 107; **Sw** 121, 124, 125

    supramammary, **O** 39, 51; **L** 107; **Sw** 121

    thoracic aortic, **Sw** 121

    tracheobronchial, **H** 27; **O** 51

    ventral thoracic, **H** 27

Lymph vessels, **H** 27; **O** 51

    chyle cistern, **H** 27; **O** 51

    intestinal trunk, **H** 27; **O** 51; **Sw** 121

    left tracheal trunk, **O** 51; **Sw** 121

    lumbar trunk, **H** 27; **O** 51; **Sw** 121

    right tracheal trunk, **H** 27

    thoracic duct, **H** 27; **O** 51; **Sw** 121

# M

Mammary glands. *See* Gland(s) and Udder

Mane, **H** 3

Manica flexoria, **L** 98

Manus (hand), **H** 3; **C** 128

Meatus, dorsal, middle, ventral, **H** 14; **O** 40; **G** 83; **L** 99; **Sw** 118

Medial canthus, **O** 32

Mesocolon, **G** 87

Mesometrium **H** 23; **O** 47

Mesosalpinx, **H** 23; **S** 69

Mesovarium, **H** 23; **O** 47; **S** 67, 69

Metacarpal tuberosity, **H** 10. *See* Bone(s)

Metacarpus, **H** 2; **O** 32, 33; **S** 54; **G** 72; **L** 90; **Sw** 111

Metatarsal cushion, **C** 128

Metatarsus, **H** 2; **O** 33; **S** 54; **G** 72; **L** 90; **Sw** 111

Milk well, **O** 33

Muscle(s)

    accessory patagial, **C** 133

    adductor, **O** 46; **S** 60; **G** 80; **L** 96, 106; **Sw** 116, 124, 125

    ascending pectoral, **H** 7; **O** 37; **S** 59; **G** 77; **L** 95; **Sw** 115

    biceps brachii, **H** 7; **O** 38; **S** 60; **G** 80; **L** 96; **Sw** 116; **C** 133

    biceps femoris, **H** 7; **Sw** 115; **C** 132, 133

    biventer. *See* Semispinalis capitis, **Sw** 117; **C** 132–135

    brachialis, **H** 7; **O** 37; **S** 59, 60; **G** 77, 80; **L** 95, 96; **Sw** 115, 116

    brachiocephalicus, **H** 7; **O** 38; **S** 59, 62; **L** 95, 101; **Sw** 115

    buccinator, **H** 7; **O** 37; **S** 59; **G** 77; **L** 95; **Sw** 115

    bulbospongiosus, **H** 20; **O** 46; **G** 84, 86; **L** 106; **Sw** 124

    bulbourethral, **Sw** 124

    caninus, **H** 7; **O** 36; **Sw** 115

    caudal capital oblique, **H** 12, 13; **O** 46; **S** 61; **G** 81; **L** 97

    caudal preputial, **O** 36; **Sw** 114

    caudal scapulohumeral, **C** 133

    cloacal elevator, **C** 132, 133

    cloacal sphincter, **C** 132, 133, 135

    coccygeus, **O** 37; **S** 60; **G** 80

    coccygeus lateralis, **C** 132, 133

    common digital extensor, **H** 7, 10; **O** 37; **S** 59; **G** 77; **L** 95; **Sw** 115

    complexus. *See* Semispinalis capitis, **Sw** 117; **C** 132–135

    cranial capital oblique, **H** 13; **O** 39; **S** 61; **G** 81; **L** 96, 97; **Sw** 116, 117

    cranial preputial, **O** 36; **Sw** 114

    cranial tibial, **H** 7, 12; **O** 37; **S** 59; **L** 95; **Sw** 115

    cutaneus colli, **H** 6; **O** 36; **S** 58; **G** 76; **L** 93; **Sw** 114; **C** 132

cutaneus faciei, **H** 6; **O** 36; **S** 58; **G** 76; **L** 93; **Sw** 114

cutaneus nasi, **G** 76

cutaneus trunci, **H** 6; **O** 36; **S** 58, 63; **G** 76; **L** 93; **Sw** 114

deep digital flexor, **H** 7, 10, 12; **O** 37, 38; **S** 59, 60; **G** 77, 80; **L** 95, 96; **Sw** 115, 116; **C** 133

deltoideus, **H** 7; **O** 37; **S** 59, 60; **G** 77, 80; **L** 95, 96; **Sw** 115; **C** 132

depressor labii inferioris, **H** 7; **S** 59; **G** 77; **Sw** 115

depressor labii superioris, **H** 7; **Sw** 115

depressor mandibulae, **C** 132

depressor palpebrae, **G** 77; **Sw** 115

descending pectoral, **H** 7; **O** 37; **G** 77; **L** 95

digastricus, **H** 12, 13

dilator naris, **H** 14

dorsal capital straight, **H** 14; **O** 39; **S** 61, **G** 81, 83; **L** 97, 99, **Sw** 119

dorsal interosseous, **C** 132

extensor carpi obliquus, **H** 7, 12; **O** 37; **S** 59; **G** 77; **L** 95; **Sw** 115

extensor carpi radialis, **H** 7, 10; **O** 37; **S** 59; **G** 77; **L** 95; **Sw** 115

extensor metacarpi radialis, **C** 132, 133

external abdominal oblique, **H** 7; **O** 37; **S** 59, 63; **G** 77; **L** 95; **Sw** 115; **C** 132, 133

external anal sphincter, **H** 20, 21; **S** 66; **Sw** 124

external mandibular adductor, **C** 132

fifth digital extensor, **Sw** 115

flexor carpi radialis, **H** 7, 10; **O** 37; **S** 59; **G** 77; **L** 95; **Sw** 115

flexor carpi ulnaris, **H** 7; **S** 59; **G** 77; **C** 133

flexor perforans and perforatus, **C** 132

frontalis, **O** 36, 37; **S** 59; **G** 77; **L** 95

frontoscutularis, **H** 6

gastrocnemius, **H** 7, 12; **O** 37, 38; **S** 59, 60; **G** 77, 80; **L** 95, 96; **Sw** 115, 116; **C** 132, 133

genioglossus, **H** 14; **G** 83; **L** 99; **Sw** 118

geniohyoideus, **H** 14; **G** 83; **L** 99; **Sw** 118

gluteobiceps, **O** 37; **S** 59; **G** 77; **L** 95

gracilis, **O** 46; **Sw** 124

hyoepiglottic, **H** 14

iliacus, **H** 12; **O** 38

iliocostalis thoracis, **H** 12; **O** 38; **S** 60; **G** 80; **L** 96; **Sw** 115, 116

infraspinatus, **H** 12; **O** 38; **S** 60; **G** 80; **L** 96

internal abdominal oblique, **H** 22; **O** 37, 47; **S** 59, 63, 66; **G** 77; **L** 95, 107

interosseus medius, **H** 10; **O** 36; **G** 78

    *See also* Suspensory ligament, **H** 7, 10, 11; **O** 37; **S** 59; **G** 77; **L** 95, 98

interosseus secundus, **L** 98

intertransversarii, **H** 12, 13; **O** 39; **S** 60, 61, 62; **G** 81; **L** 95, 96, 97; **Sw** 116, 117

intertransversarius longus, **O** 38; **S** 61; **G** 81; **L** 97

ischiocavernosus, **O** 46; **S** 64, 66; **G** 84, 86; **L** 104, 106; **Sw** 124

lateral digital extensor, **H** 7, 10, 12; **O** 37; **S** 59; **G** 77; **L** 95; **Sw** 115

latissimus dorsi, **H** 7; **O** 37; **S** 59; **G** 77; **L** 95; **Sw** 115; **C** 132, 133

levator ani, **C** 132, 133

levator coccygeus, **C** 132, 133

levator labii superioris, **H** 7; **O** 36; **Sw** 115

levator nasolabialis, **H** 7; **O** 36; **S** 59; **G** 77; **L** 95; **Sw** 115

long digital extensor, **H** 7, 12; **O** 37; **S** 59; **G** 77; **L** 95

long patagial tensor, **C** 132, 133

longissimus atlantis, **H** 12; **O** 38; **S** 60; **G** 80; **L** 95; **Sw** 116, 117

longissimus capitis, **H** 12; **O** 38; **S** 60; **G** 80; **L** 95, 96; **Sw** 116, 117

longissimus cervicis, **H** 12; **O** 38; **S** 60; **G** 80; **L** 95, 96; **Sw** 117

longissimus thoracis and lumborum, **H** 12; **O** 38; **S** 60; **G** 80; **L** 96; **Sw** 116

longus atlantis, **L** 96

longus capitis, **H** 12, 14; **S** 60; **G** 80; **L** 96, 99; **Sw** 116, 117

longus coli, **H** 12, 14; **S** 61, 62; **G** 81, 83; **L** 97, 99, 101; **C** 133, 134, 135

major long digital flexor, **C** 133

malaris, **O** 37; **S** 59; **G** 77

masseter, **H** 7; **O** 37; **S** 59, 62; **G** 77; **L** 95; **Sw** 115

mentalis, **H** 14; **Sw** 115

middle gluteal, **H** 7, 19; **O** 37, 38; **S** 59, 60; **G** 77, 80; **L** 95, 96; **Sw** 115, 116

multifidus cervicis, **H** 13; **O** 39; **S** 61; **G** 80, 81; **L** 97

mylohyoideus, **O** 37

obturator internis, **H** 23; **O** 46, 47

occipital hyoideus, **H** 12

omohyoideus, **H** 7, 14; **S** 62

omotransversarius, **H** 7; **O** 37; **S** 59; **G** 77; **L** 95; **Sw** 115

orbicularis oris, **Sw** 115

parotidoauricularis, **H** 7; **S** 59, 62; **G** 77; **L** 95

peroneus longus, **O** 37; **S** 59; **G** 77; **L** 95; **Sw** 115; **C** 132, 133

peroneus tertius, **H** 7, 11; **O** 37; **S** 59; **G** 77; **L** 95; **Sw** 115

platysma, **Sw** 114

psoas major, **O** 38; **Sw** 116

quadratus lumborum, **Sw** 116

quadriceps femoris, **H** 11, 12

rectus abdominis, **H** 22; **S** 66, 67; **G** 86, 87; **L** 106, 107; **Sw** 124, 125

rectus femoris, **H** 12; **O** 38; **S** 60; **G** 80; **L** 96; **Sw** 116

retractor penis, **H** 20; **O** 44, 46; **S** 64, 66; **G** 84, 86; **L** 106; **Sw** 124

rhomboideus, **H** 7, 12; **O** 38; **S** 60; **G** 80; **L** 96; **Sw** 116; **C** 134

sacrocaudalis, **O** 37

sartorius, **C** 132, 133

scalenus, **H** 12; **O** 38, 39; **S** 60; **G** 80; **L** 96, 101

scutularis, **O** 36

semimembranosus, **H** 7, 12; **O** 38; **S** 59, 60; **G** 80; **L** 95, 96; **Sw** 115, 116; **C** 132, 133

semispinalis capitis, **H** 12; **S** 60; **G** 80; **Sw** 117, 118

    biventer cervicis, **Sw** 117; **C** 132, 133, 134, 135

    complexus, **Sw** 117; **C** 132–135

semitendinosus, **H** 7, 12; **O** 37, 38; **S** 59, 60; **G** 80; **L** 95, 96; **Sw** 115; **C** 132, 133

serratus dorsalis caudalis, **H** 7; **O** 35

serratus dorsalis cranialis, **G** 77; **L** 95

serratus superficialis, **C** 133

serratus ventralis, **H** 7; **O** 37; **S** 59; **G** 77; **L** 95, 96; **Sw** 115, 116

short digital extensor, **H** 12; **Sw** 115

Penis—*Continued*
    spongy tubercle, **S** 68
Peritoneal cavity, **S** 63
Peritoneum. *See* Serosa, **S** 63
Pes, **H** 2
Phallic bodies. *See* Cloaca
Pharynx, **C** 136
    laryngopharynx, **O** 40; **G** 83; **L** 99; **Sw** 118
    nasopharynx, **H** 14; **O** 40; **G** 83; **L** 99; **Sw** 118
    oropharynx, **H** 14; **O** 40; **G** 83; **L** 99; **Sw** 118
    pharyngeal recess, **Sw** 118
    pharyngeal septum, **O** 40; **G** 83
    pharyngeal tonsil, **G** 83
Pin, **O** 32
Pinna, **H** 3; **O** 32, 33; **S** 54, 59; **G** 72, 73; **L** 90, 91
Point
    of elbow, **H** 2; **O** 32; **G** 73; **L** 91; **Sw** 110
    of hip, **H** 3; **Sw** 111
    of hock, **H** 3; **O** 33; **S** 55; **G** 73; **L** 91; **Sw** 110
    of shoulder, **H** 2; **O** 32; **G** 73; **L** 91; **Sw** 111
Poll, **H** 2; **O** 32, 33; **G** 72, 73; **L** 90; **Sw** 111
Pouch(es)
    cutaneous, **S** 54, 55
    guttural, **H** 14
Preen gland. *See* Gland(s), uropygial
Prepuce, **H** 2, 22; **S** 54, 68; **G** 76, 86; **L** 106; **Sw** 110, 114, 124
    external (sheath), **H** 22
    internal, **H** 22; **S** 68
    preputial diverticulum, **Sw** 114, 124
    preputial orifice, **O** 32; **S** 124
Proctodeum. *See* Cloaca
Propatagium, **C** 128, 129
Proventriculus, **C** 135, 136, 138, 139
Pygostyle. *See* Bone(s)
Pylorus. *See* Stomach

### Q

Quarter, **H** 2

### R

Rack, **S** 56
Reciprocal apparatus, **H** 11
Rectum, **H** 16, 20, 21, 23; **O** 41, 45, 46, 47; **S** 61, 65, 66, 67; **G** 80, 84, 86, 87; **L** 103, 105, 106, 107; **Sw** 117, 123, 124, 125; **C** 134, 136, 138, 139, 140, 141
    ampulla, **H** 23
    transverse plicae, **H** 22
Reticulum, **O** 39, 41, 43, 45; **S** 64, 65; **G** 85
Rib margin. *See* Bone(s)
Round, **O** 32
Rumen, **O** 39, 42, 43, 45; **S** 60, 61, 63, 64, 65; **G** 81, 84, 85
    interior, **O** 41; **S** 63
Rump, **O** 32; **S** 54; **G** 72; **L** 90; **Sw** 110

### S

Saddle, **C** 128, 130
Scrotum, **H** 22; **O** 32, 38; **S** 54, 66; **G** 86; **L** 106; **Sw** 110, 114
    seminal vesicle. *See* Gland(s)
    tunica albuginea, **S** 58; **G** 76
Serosa of rumen, **S** 63
Shank, **C** 128, 129
Shoulder, **H** 3; **O** 32; **S** 54, 56; **G** 72; **L** 90; **Sw** 110; **C** 128, 129
Sinus
    frontal, **H** 14; **O** 40; **G** 83, 84; **L** 99; **Sw** 118
    cornual diverticulum, **O** 44; **G** 84
    sphenoid, **H** 14; **Sw** 118
Skin & subcutis, **S** 63; **G** 79
Slipper, **L** 91, 98
Snout, **Sw** 110, 111
Spermatic cord, **H** 22; **Sw** 122, 124
Spinal cord, **H** 14, 28, 29; **O** 50; **G** 83; **L** 99; **Sw** 118
Spleen, **H** 13, 19, 21; **O** 39, 43, 45, 51; **S** 61; **G** 81; **L** 97; **Sw** 117, 123; **C** 138, 139
Spur, **C** 128
Stay apparatus
    forelimb, **H** 10
    hindlimb, **H** 11
Sternocoracoclavicular membrane, **C** 134

femoral, **H** 26; **O** 48
hepatic, **H** 26; **O** 48
iliolumbar, **H** 26
intercostal, **H** 26; **O** 48; **Sw** 123
internal iliac, **H** 26; **O** 48
internal jugular, **O** 48; **S** 62
internal thoracic, **H** 26; **O** 48
interosseous, **O** 48
jugular, **L** 95, 101, 104, 105; **C** 132, 133, 134, 135, 139
lateral auricular, **Sw** 114
lateral palmar, **H** 26
lateral plantar, **O** 48
lateral sacral, **H** 26
lateral saphenous, **H** 7, 26; **O** 37, 48; **S** 59; **G** 77
lateral thoracic, **H** 7; **Sw** 114
linguofacial, **H** 26; **G** 77
maxillary, **H** 26; **O** 48; **S** 62; **G** 77
medial plantar, **H** 26; **O** 48
medial saphenous, **H** 26; **O** 48; **S** 59; **G** 77
median, **H** 26; **O** 37, 48
median sacral, **O** 48
milk. *See* Subcutaneous abdominal, **O** 33, 36, 37; **G** 73, 77
occipital, **H** 26; **O** 48; **S** 62
ovarian, **H** 26
palmar common digital, **O** 48
palmar proper digital, **O** 48
pampiniform plexus, **O** 46; **S** 66; **G** 86; **L** 106
plantar common digital, **O** 48
plantar proper digital, **O** 48
popliteal, **O** 48
portal, **O** 48
prostatic, **H** 26; **O** 48
pudendal epigastric, **H** 26; **O** 48
pulmonary, **H** 25; **O** 45; **S** 65; **G** 85; **L** 105; **C** 138

radial, **S** 59; **G** 77
renal, **H** 26; **O** 48
rostral auricular, **H** 26
subclavian, **H** 26; **O** 48; **S** 65; **G** 85
subcutaneous abdominal, **O** 33, 37; **G** 73, 77
subscapular, **H** 26; **O** 48
superficial cervical, **H** 26; **O** 48
superficial thoracic, **H** 26
testicular, **H** 22, 26; **O** 46, 48; **S** 66; **G** 86; **L** 106; **Sw** 124
thoracodorsal, **H** 26; **O** 48
transverse facial, **H** 26
umbilical, **H** 24
vertebral, **H** 26, **O** 48
Vent, **C** 132, 134, 135, 140
Ventriculus (gizzard), **C** 134, 135, 136, 138, 139
Vulva, **H** 13, 21, 23; **O** 45, 47; **S** 65; **G** 73, 77, 85; **L** 105; **Sw** 117, 123, 125
clitoris, **H** 23; **O** 47; **S** 67; **L** 107
vulvar labia, **H** 23; **O** 47; **S** 67, 69; **G** 87; **L** 107

## W

Wattle(s), **G** 73; **C** 128, 129
Wing bar. *See* Feather(s)
Wing bow. *See* Feather(s)
Withers, **H** 2; **O** 32; **S** 54; **G** 72; **L** 90; **Sw** 111
Wrist joint. *See* Joint(s)

## X

Xiphoid process. *See* Bone(s), sternum

## Z

Zygomatic arch, **H** 13. *See also* Bone(s)